Timely Psychosocial Interventions
in Dementia Care

Timely Psychosocial Interventions in Dementia Care

Evidence-Based Practice

Edited by **Jill Manthorpe** and **Esme Moniz-Cook**

Foreword by **Helen Rochford-Brennan,**
Chairperson of the European Working Group of
People with Dementia

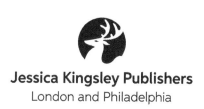

Jessica Kingsley Publishers
London and Philadelphia

First published in 2020
by Jessica Kingsley Publishers
73 Collier Street
London N1 9BE, UK
and
400 Market Street, Suite 400
Philadelphia, PA 19106, USA

www.jkp.com

Library of Congress Cataloging in Publication Data
A CIP catalog record for this book is available from the Library of Congress

British Library Cataloguing in Publication Data
A CIP catalogue record for this book is available from the British Library

ISBN 9781 78775 302 0
eISBN 9781 78775 303 7

Printed and bound in Great Britain

Contents

Foreword

It's with immense gratitude and pleasure that I welcome this book as it resonates with me and many others with the illness. I am delighted the conversation about the importance of social health and psychosocial interventions has seriously started.

As a person with dementia my social health is very important to my daily life. When I was diagnosed social health was never discussed with me. I was much more aware of social disengagement as sadly nobody within the health sector explained to me I could carry on with my daily life and engagement with my community. I was grieving for a life I would never have; I was not offered any post diagnostic support due to my age. I forgot I had rights and should be treated like everyone else and be fully integrated into my community as an equal citizen.

My personhood was never discussed with me, or how I could be empowered or supported, or my anxiety could be lessened by having activities. I had to cope with a new language – being 'demented' and 'dementia friendly communities' – which heighted my anxiety. I was very aware I had rights under the United Nations Convention on Rights of Persons with Disabilities and all I required was adjustment, not another title. I was offered medication which had horrendous side effects.

Thanks to my involvement with Public and Patient Involvement in Research, I was able to access cognitive rehabilitative therapy which gave me the tools to cope with my memory deficit. Finally, I was being enabled not disenabled. I was learning new skills or relearning old ones. I could support my family with the school and sports runs, use technology which gave me a sense of pride, develop my rose garden and walk daily to ensure I had outdoor activities.

Today with support like this I live a very meaningful life, full of joy and good relationships. I have a sense of purpose which gives me a good quality of life. This also impacts on my family and community who acknowledge my brain disease.

Timely psychosocial interventions would have changed my life. Today, as Chair of the European Working Group of People with Dementia, it's a privilege for me to promote our rights to psychosocial interventions from the time of diagnosis and beyond.

Helen Rochford-Brennan
Chairperson of the European Working
Group of People with Dementia –
EWGPWD

Chapter 1

Timely Support for People with Dementia

NEW AGENDAS AND CHALLENGES

Jill Manthorpe and Esme Moniz-Cook

Introduction

Dementia has come of age. Most developed countries now have a national dementia strategy and there is a Global Dementia Council. It is a condition known about and feared by the public. In the United Kingdom (UK), dementia-friendly communities and dementia friends are novel social movements aimed at inspiring the public to offer support to people with dementia whom they don't know. Numbers are being addressed with greater confidence and modelling is being undertaken to estimate population trends (Ahmadi-Abhari *et al.* 2017). This is a very different context from our earlier book on psychosocial interventions, where telling people about dementia was often the professional task. One challenge for professionals is to prevent or minimise disability and distress particularly around the time of diagnosis, but also to identify their own roles and skills in supporting people affected by dementia during the months or years that they have to live with the condition. There is greater humility amongst professionals about whether they know all the answers; indeed there is increasing recognition that professional education is not always fit for purpose (Surr *et al.* 2017).

The idea of 'prescribed disengagement' has been gaining ground in criticisms of current dementia practice (Swaffer 2015). Defined as a process that at the time of diagnosis 'sets up a chain reaction of defeat and fear, which negatively impacts a person's ability to be positive, resilient and proactive' (Swaffer 2015, p.3), ways to counteract this are relevant to many practice settings. People with dementia are inspiring such approaches (Mitchell 2018; Swaffer 2015). Although the recent review by Low *et al.* (2018) did not find direct evidence for prescribed disengagement, the contribution of diagnostic and post-diagnostic processes to disempowerment of the person with dementia, and exacerbation of negative views or self-stigma around dementia, are acknowledged. The term appears to have found traction within dementia communities, suggesting that practitioners need to be aware that other people may regard them as promoting disengagement. The new professional task may be to actively prove otherwise.

The concept of 'social health' as one way to challenge these negative discourses has prompted a new research agenda (Vernooij-Dassen and Jeon 2016). This may also stimulate new approaches to practice, education and skill development. Dröes *et al.* (2017) suggest that promoting social health for people with dementia has to take into account the following factors: 'personal' (e.g. sense of coherence; competencies); 'disease-related' (e.g. severity of cognitive impairment; comorbidity); 'social' (e.g. network support; stigma) and 'environmental' (e.g. 'enabling' design; accessibility). In many ways this resembles the changes demanded by the disability movement, who challenge the medical model of pathology and paternalism.

Background: Timely psychosocial interventions

In the opening chapter of this book we use six anonymised case illustrations to demonstrate how, at the time of diagnosis and beyond, ideas of 'prescribed disengagement' and social health may relate to the particular circumstances of people affected by dementia, and how they can be used as frameworks for optimised practice and service design.

In this section we present the background to our arguments that 'timely dementia interventions' need to spread beyond the diagnostic and immediate post-diagnostic period. Much UK research has identified the gap between dementia diagnosis and any support for the process of adjustment (Campbell *et al.* 2016) but this has not always acknowledged that timely interventions are lacking across the dementia trajectory. Therefore, this book illustrates practice for people affected by dementia and their families in home care settings (Chapters 2–11) as well as those living in care homes supported by paid staff (Chapters 12–18).

As with our earlier book, the lack of attention to the impacts of early dementia on family members and others in the social network remains. Until they take up the tasks of 'caring', family members stay rather 'shadowy' in both research and practice. Social networks, particularly families, are an important part of the social context for people with dementia and the impact of a psychosocial intervention will be influenced by this context across the dementia trajectory. Therefore, the person and people close to them, including supporting family and friends, will all need to engage with the aims of psychosocial intervention. In order to properly focus an intervention, we need to consider the personal circumstances, relationships, concerns and hopes of both the person with dementia and their family (Chapter 2).

The conceptual and empirical basis of early intervention programmes in dementia care is underpinned by models of psychosocial support for disability and psychosocial wellbeing. The aims of psychosocial interventions may also be set within the paradigm of health promotion, which broadly reflects the notion of social health. The three dimensions of social health applied to dementia include '(i) capacity to fulfil potential and obligations; (ii) ability to manage life with some degree of independence; and (iii) participation in social activities' (Dröes *et al.* 2017, p.4). For each dimension there will be influencing factors and effective interventions, but there is still much to learn. For example, little is known about whether and how 'secondary health promoting interventions' can maintain wellbeing, or delay the progressive disabilities of a long-term condition, or act on symptom-control. In working with people with early dementia, the aims of 'secondary health promoting interventions' may be to:

- prevent future distress by addressing the longer term sources of 'excess disabilities' (i.e. the extra health and psychosocial disabilities commonly encountered by people with dementia that are not directly related to brain damage or cognitive loss)

- promote maintenance of purpose, pleasure, meaningful activity, valued relationships and quality of life.

Therefore the prophylactic function of interventions that have strategies for preventing distress and disability and promoting health and psychosocial wellbeing is implicit within our defined aims of *timely intervention in dementia*. Furthermore, interventions may be offered irrespective of a dementia diagnosis, including when this is uncertain, where a 'watching brief' is needed, or where Mild Cognitive Impairment (MCI) is present, or at the end of life, when dementia may not be the major presenting problem and comfort is needed for all concerned. Three particular areas are therefore explored:

- health promotion
- pre-empting negative reactions
- supporting people affected by dementia.

Health promotion

In recent years the notion of 'preventable dementia' has arisen with epidemiological studies of risk factors,[1] neuro-protection and neuronal reserve enhancement (Livingston *et al.* 2017). The global World Wide FINGERS network[2] launched in 2017 is a research initiative with multiple trials underway seeking to prevent or delay cognitive decline, confirming this rising interest. Cautious evidence-based claims are being made that some future cases of dementia can be prevented, with estimates being given for specific populations. The British Psychological Society (2018) estimated that up to one third of cases of Alzheimer's disease were attributable to 'the effects of potentially-modifiable factors, such as diabetes, midlife hypertension, midlife obesity, physical inactivity, depression, smoking and limited educational opportunity early in life' (p.5). It recommended that social initiatives should target inequality and deprivation, increase activity and improve general health and fitness in the population, to potentially reduce the prevalence of dementia.

From this literature the treatment of vascular risk factors, such as hypertension, diabetes, high cholesterol, narrowing of the main arteries to the brain, heart disease and smoking, are all identified as important preventative strategies, and these continue to apply to many people with dementia, aimed at maintenance of physical wellbeing. Similarly, strategies for protection in the prevention of further damage – such as treatment for levels of folate and vitamin B12 or antioxidants (vitamins C and E and alcohol), may be equally applicable after a dementia diagnosis.

---

1   See www.thelancet.com/infographics/dementia2017
2   http://wwfingers.com

There is an emerging empirical basis for psychosocial intervention in preventing dementia-related disabilities, described as proactive re-enablement (Poulos *et al.* 2017). This may include physical activity, cognitive rehabilitation (Chapter 7) and family support (see Case Study 1.5 'Darren and Julie' below).

Since the our first book on psychosocial interventions, the overall potential for prevention (Livingston *et al.* 2017) is far more comprehensive and better evidenced. The health-promotion literature outlines risks to functional independence, health and wellbeing in older people, including medication effects and injurious falls. A health promotion strategy for dementia may therefore include:

- monitoring the known risk factors, including hearing loss (Livingston *et al.* 2017), of developing further dementia symptoms and provided timely treatment when needed

- addressing known risks, such as loneliness (Sutin *et al.* 2018), falls (Sharma *et al.* 2018) and through medicine management (Maidment *et al.* 2017)

- keeping in touch (monitoring) with people with dementia and carers, providing psychosocial interventions when needed and acceptable (such as cognitive, physical, social and pleasurable activity) to maintain psychosocial wellbeing or social health.

Pre-empting negative reactions

The powerful impact of the double stigma of age and dementia needs to be acknowledged. Patterson *et al.* (2018) describe the negative social experiences that people with dementia can encounter where a sense of being treated as an 'other' or a 'lesser being' exacerbates social pathology. For many older people stigma brings with it fears of loss of control and prompts misunderstandings of what can be achieved to minimise or postpone distress and disability. This can have a subtle but important effect on the potential for older people and their families to engage with health-promoting and psychosocial interventions that may help protect against the known negative consequences of a dementia on wellbeing and quality of life.

Some practices undermine engagement of older people and families in programmes to promote health and psychosocial wellbeing. For example, some protocols of pre-diagnostic counselling require a person to decide whether they wish to be told their diagnosis or not. As they may have only just tentatively decided that it is worth exploring what is on offer to overcome as yet unexpressed fears, this may be inappropriate (Moniz-Cook *et al.* 2006). These may reinforce fears of loss of control. Post-diagnostic protocols for acetylcholinesterase inhibitor (AChEI) medications, information on matters such as Lasting Power of Attorney (appointment of a chosen proxy in England and Wales), Advance Decisions ('living wills'), social security benefits, continence, driving, safety and signposting to local and national organisations have their place, but they can sometimes undermine active engagement in proactive collaborative psychosocial interventions, particularly if they are overwhelming, and may be viewed as forms of 'prescribed disengagement'. Where clinical services have been established primarily for evaluation of AChEI medications and these are not suitable for an individual, other forms of protective interventions may be rejected by disappointed family carers or under-resourced, skill-deficient practitioners and protocols. Finally, if family anxieties are not addressed at the start, relatives may inadvertently undermine or not actively support activities that promote health and wellbeing. For some, coping by oneself may seem a 'safe' option.

A psychosocial dementia care model is primarily asset-based, where approaches should focus on remaining abilities and attend to the use of language to avoid negative stereotyping (again reflecting the risk of 'prescribed disengagement'). They can promote activity of choice, autonomy and normalise personalised activity-support (reflecting the concept of social health), by basing this on knowledge of current or past pleasures, values and interests. Such a model can also have a gatekeeping function to prevent others – such as families and practitioners – from undermining access to interventions, for example on the grounds that they are too risky or inappropriate. Ways of attending to this could involve:

- neutralising stigma at the time of assessment and later professional encounters (see illustrative case studies)

- promoting social health and psychosocial wellbeing (Vernooij-Dassen, Moniz-Cook and Jeon 2018) in goal assessment and care planning

- supporting family members to access help (Vernooij-Dassen and Jeon 2016).

Within the UK NHS context a person with dementia will generally be 'case managed' in primary care by the person's GP unless the person moves to long-term care where the care home staff take on many coordinating roles. A minority of people are referred on to specialist mental health services, though many eventually make use of publicly funded social care services to some extent and are in contact with local authorities. However, there are problems of service capacity; in England community-based teams working with older people with mental health problems may have limited capacity to take on work with people living at home whose behaviour is distressing (Manthorpe *et al.* 2018), because other referrals have greater priority. This means that primary and social care practitioners have to draw on their own skills repertoire and experience. While talking of the potential for psychosocial interventions, it is important to acknowledge that social care for people with dementia and others is often very limited, arriving 'too little and too late' (Age UK 2018); resources are limited in other countries too. Dementia stakeholders, while advocating for investment in care services, can argue that it is all the more important to focus on remaining abilities and avoid negative stereotyping to postpone care needs by:

- clarifying the person's strengths and how these may be maximised

- providing compensatory strategies for particular difficulties due to cognitive loss.

The following two case illustrations describe how an asset-based approach to intervention at the time of diagnosis may minimise the impact of negative stereotyping and guide timely intervention.

Case Study 1.1 – **Jenny**

Jenny, aged 82, attended the memory clinic because her husband, Gregory, was convinced that she had Alzheimer's disease and wanted her to take any drugs (i.e. the AChEIs) that might help. Jenny herself was not keen on any drugs – *'let alone drugs for the mind'*. She felt that her memory *'was fine'*. The couple had gone on the internet to find out about dementia, before attending the clinic.

15

They both agreed that in the past three months Jenny had become hesitant and lacking in confidence, particularly with housework. Gregory felt that he now had to do more round the home. Jenny had also recently decided to stop driving. Following initial assessment, Jenny declined a brain scan (MRI) for diagnostic clarification. A working diagnosis of Mild Cognitive Impairment was discussed with them. Gregory was upset that 'nothing could be done'. Having outlined her day-to-day concerns, Jenny requested, and was given, a written summary of the meeting for her to share with their daughter who lived elsewhere. Their daughter travelled to attend a half-day workshop with Jenny on 'Understanding and managing memory problems'.

By maintaining internet communication with her parents most days, the daughter encouraged her father to provide day-to-day support, including in-home strategies to help compensate for Jenny's memory difficulties. Gregory continued to feel that Jenny would benefit from medication, but his daughter encouraged him to help Jenny in her efforts to maintain her pleasurable activities. He joined a local choir with her. Eighteen months later Jenny was diagnosed at the memory clinic with a mixed Alzheimer's/vascular-type dementia. Gregory continued to want Jenny to take up the offer of an AChEI, but she maintained that she did not want to 'take drugs for the mind'. She attended a seven-week group cognitive stimulation therapy course (see Chapter 5) at the memory clinic and continued with her choir and an art class.

Shortly after the dementia diagnosis, a memory clinic assistant successfully encouraged Jenny and Gregory to use the internet to locate and join a fortnightly dance activity, since they had previously enjoyed dancing at parties and charity functions. A year later their daughter (who now was in telephone contact with the healthcare assistant) reported that her parents were relatively active and had made new friends at their dance sessions, whom they met occasionally for coffee or lunch. Gregory was still keen that Jenny should try an anti-dementia drug but she continued to say no.

Case Study 1.1 reflects how the risk of disengagement was present even before the initial clinic visit but was managed. Social health, in the form of activities that both partners may attend, is described, but so too the important supportive role of their daughter and, later, the timely brief support from a healthcare assistant. Engagement with the internet is also changing the professional–patient relationship.

Recommendations about reliable personally relevant information with timely encouragement, and support to remain active, may be part of the professional 'offer'.

Case Study 1.2 – **Sally**

Sally, aged 68, had lived with her daughter Brenda for the last 20 years, helping her in childcare and managing the home. Sally confessed to the practice nurse that she was concerned about her memory. Brenda did not feel that her mother had memory problems but thought she had become increasingly 'lazy' and had lost interest in the house. She felt that she had to constantly 'nag' at her mother to do things. They both agreed that this was leading to increasing tension.

A memory assessment indicated that Sally was developing 'dysexecutive syndrome', where more than one of the cognitive deficits associated with the front of the brain was noted, including difficulties with task initiation. In contrast, most aspects of memory function were relatively unimpaired. A functional diagram of the brain was used to explain to Sally and Brenda the consequences of everyday behavioural deficits associated with 'dysexecutive syndrome'. These included the 'sharpness of tongue' and 'rudeness' that Brenda said was unusual for Sally, and how reduced 'initiation' can affect a person's ability to do what they want to do. Brenda remained sceptical and decided to await the outcome of an MRI scan, which was under way.

In the meantime she and her mother attended the half-day workshop where Jenny and her daughter (see Jenny 'Case Study 1.1') were also present. They had understood the concept of difficulty in initiating tasks due to 'starter motor problems' and described their successes in overcoming the effects of this through trial and error of what worked for Jenny, using the advice provided. This motivated Brenda to take advantage of rehabilitation techniques to prompt initiation and thus assist her mother in increasing her activity around the home. Subsequently Sally was diagnosed with a frontal-type dementia that progressed rapidly but the mother–daughter relationship remained close and had not suffered from Brenda's early feelings of exasperation with her mother.

Case Study 1.2 demonstrates how the risk of disengagement has potential to escalate into conflict. The relationship between mother and daughter benefited from information and advice, and from discovering how others were managing.

Promoting control and pleasure

Several of the interventions described in this book are designed to enhance neuronal reserves through cognitive, social and leisure activity. In early dementia, such interventions can have two separate aims:

- to provide cognition-orientated activity that promotes a sense of control and autonomy by counteracting the anxieties and fears (Moniz-Cook *et al.* 2006) associated with declining memory in ageing

- to promote normalisation and social integration in the form of purposeful, meaningful activity and friendships, since these are core components of positive mental health and wellbeing and have long been known as moderators of hopelessness and depression in later life (Takahashi, Tamura and Tokoro 1997).

Arts-based activities are often well-received examples of engagement, and recent work is improving understandings of what might be essential attributes of their effectiveness. Windle *et al.* (2017) suggest that stimulating aesthetic experiences and dynamic and responsive artistic practice can lead to benefits for people with conditions across the dementia spectrum and are important for cognitive, social and individual responses. Such characteristics may also be found in activities such as making or listening to music or dance (Chapters 12 and 13).

Supporting people affected by dementia

Approaches to cognitive rehabilitation can include advice on maximising cognitive strengths. These can be encouraged during conversation, activities of daily living and leisure, or individualised cognitive rehabilitation. 'Prophylactic cognitive rehabilitation' (a rather complicated term) involves general use of external memory aids. Examples include technology-based reminders (Chapter 9) or use of 'orientation/white boards', automatic calendars and notebooks. These are used to help establish implicit orientation procedures to counteract future decline in prospective and episodic memory. Rehabilitation often includes the person's family or friends who wish to help. The case study of Nitan illustrates how the wider care network may also support use of external memory aides.

Case Study 1.3 – **Nitan**

Nitan, a retired accountant aged 77, had moved from the Indian subcontinent to the UK. His sense of pride lay in his excellent memory, which despite his early dementia did not initially cause him or his wife problems. He resisted engagement in cognitive rehabilitation to establish implicit orientation procedures, since he believed that this would be the 'lazy way out' and that he needed to 'stimulate his memory by testing it each day'. In his opinion a cognitive rehabilitation programme would only be necessary if and when his memory worsened.

Six months later Nitan was feeling 'under the weather' and was seen by his family doctor (GP). During this consultation Nitan discovered that his GP, whose opinion he valued, used memory aids to improve his own memory efficacy. Encouraged by his GP, and with support from his wife and a dementia adviser, Nitan engaged in memory training using external memory aides of his choice (in his case using a notebook of a type that he had used at work). Nitan lived at home with his wife for two further years, until he required two months of palliative care during the final stages of cancer.

Individualised cognitive rehabilitation usually involves active learning to compensate for, or resolve, current everyday concerns for the person, or more often problems reported by adult children whose parent lives alone, such as repeated questioning and seemingly demanding phone calls (Evans, Price and Meyer 2016). Individualised cognitive rehabilitation requires targeted support from a therapist with knowledge of learning methods, such as spaced-retrieval and errorless learning. Rehabilitation is usually tailored to the person to support them to achieve their own goals in a relatively short period of time (Chapters 6 and 7). The case study of Charles illustrates how people living alone can be helped to overcome their memory-related problems and live at home. It reminds us that not all social networks are conducive to wellbeing.

Case Study 1.4 – **Charles**

Charles, aged 64, had recently allowed into his home teenage boys known to experiment with drugs. His son and neighbours were concerned as Charles insisted on keeping money at home. He was a friendly man who was generous to other young people such as his nieces and nephews. Charles was also an active man and relatively independent; apart from support with food preparation and laundry from his housing provider, he looked after himself despite his early onset dementia. In his view a move to a care home for his safety was not an option as *'he would rather be dead, like his brother who had dementia'*. His brother had apparently survived only two months following a care home move some years previously.

As part of a multi-agency safeguarding plan to protect him from abuse, a face-recognition programme was established with the cooperation of his neighbour and a nephew using six familiar people and six 'stooge strangers' who initially visited him at home each day, and photo-recognition was added to his mobile phone. The frequency of visits was graded over eight weeks until he consistently refused entry to strangers over three consecutive weeks. His home care team continued to monitor that Charles was no longer at risk of exploitation from local drug misusers or others. He lived at home until his death of a heart attack, some four years later.

In Case Study 1.4, the support plan needed to involve agencies that were wider than healthcare, emphasising the social model of support. For other people affected by dementia, maximising cognitive strengths using the principles of compensation (making up for problems in one area by enhancing other features) may be more relevant. Strategies include applying focused attention techniques, reducing cognitive load and maintaining pleasurable mental activity. Examples of these in communication are: using short sentences or closed questions and avoiding pronouns during conversation; reducing the demand for sustained conversation during activities of daily living, such as during domestic activities and at mealtimes; enhancing memory retrieval using errorless learning with visual and verbal cues, taking care not to 'test' the person's failing memory when forgetting is obvious; and developing personal plans for pleasurable activity that are based on past interest and values and are also achievable. Several of the following chapters illustrate these in practice in home settings (Chapters 3, 6, 7,

8 and 9), care homes (Chapters 12–18) and meeting places (Chapters 4, 5, 10 and 11).

Purposeful, pleasurable and social activity

Creative ways to support people with dementia and their spouses or partners to engage in or maintain activities that have value, meaning and purpose and provide pleasure have been the hallmark of psychosocial interventions over the past decade. They can have two separate aims:

- to maintain quality of life through engagement and participation

- to prevent or treat mood disorders in people with dementia and/ or their family carers.

As Chapter 5 shows, people with dementia and their family members find pleasure in a wide range of activities, just like anyone else. Their wide-ranging scope (also relevant to the notion of 'social health') is outlined in Chapter 6. Examples of personal pleasurable activity can be housework or homemaking, going for walks or to a leisure centre, going on holiday, regular singing and dancing sessions with friends, listening to or playing music, joining in quizzes, using a computer or phone, and sharing meals with friends. Examples of contributing to others and acts of citizenship include volunteering (Chapter 6), looking after grandchildren, baking for neighbours, talking to newly diagnosed people with dementia and fund raising, and new opportunities to take part in dementia self-advocacy and empowerment (Mitchell 2018; Swaffer 2015). The role of voluntary (third sector), community and faith groups has become central to asset-based work (SCIE 2011), and skills in community development may need to be prioritised in the dementia workforce of the future.

It has long been recognised that depression coexists in people with dementia and their family carer (Teri and Truax 1994). Engaging in and maintaining pleasurable activity and social contact have been emphasised as key ingredients of traditional behavioural activation and counselling interventions that directly aim to prevent or manage mood disorder among people with dementia and families (Chapters 8 and 10) and people in care homes (Chapter 14). Additionally, this book includes a variety of interventions that are relevant to improving or maintaining mental health among people and families at home (Chapters 3 and 11) and in care homes (Chapters 13, 15, 16 and 17). These approaches have components that: facilitate social interaction; schedule enjoyable and valued activities; involve a spouse, partner or friend in the activity for shared pleasure; or modify these approaches for people living alone (Evans *et al.* 2016); offer structure and new opportunities where these do not exist; and provide resources such as transport or volunteers to support the activity where needed.

Timely psychosocial support for managing mood and other dementia-related problems as they arise can be part of monitoring or 'keeping in touch' with people and carers. This is demonstrated in the next case illustration about Darren who was discharged from a memory clinic following his dementia diagnosis. He had felt that he was '*not that bad*' but had attended the clinic because his wife had been concerned about him. This time he was referred by the GP, because his wife was concerned that Darren's '*dementia had deteriorated*'; she was having trouble coping with him.

Case Study 1.5 – **Darren and Julie**

Darren, aged 83, had been diagnosed with Alzheimer's disease some five years ago and had maintained a relatively active life until a year ago. His wife, Julie, reported that he had become clumsy, often knocking tea cups over, he was unsteady on his feet, often stumbling and holding on to furniture to feel safe. Following hospitalisation after a fall whilst out with his rambling club a year ago, Darren was fearful of falling again. He had lost confidence in doing things at home, when tending to his garden, or going out. Julie believed that he was now too frail to engage in many activities. The consequence was that he was feeling depressed.

An assessment by the community nurse suggested he had new difficulties with depth perception and Darren's strengths and specific dementia-related cognitive weaknesses were discussed with him and Julie. This covered reasons for some of the functional problems they had been experiencing for some years, and the recent changes in the last year that were having a negative impact on their life. Once reassured, Darren and Julie engaged in a re-enablement programme to compensate for these problems.

Darren attended a six-week course at a gym, prescribed by his GP, and Julie helped by driving him there each week. Cognitive rehabilitation (Chapter 7) involved them working on goals to maintain Darren's autonomy and pleasure, for example using strategies to overcome his 'clumsiness', using equipment to prevent falls and to reassure Julie (a walking aid and wrist-watch technology to call for help if needed); and a staged programme of accompanied walking. Darren resumed going out for his daily newspaper and doing some gardening, taking regular walks around the village on his own. Later Darren and Julie joined a local walking group, where they met new people, one of whom invited Darren to a gardening discussion club, which he enjoyed. Six months on, Darren reported that he was now much happier in himself. Nonetheless, Julie remained worried about him, requiring ongoing access to, and reassurance from, the community nurse. She often felt that her husband whom she 'loved and relied on' was 'not himself'.

In this case study, the risk of disengagement is addressed by considering fears, providing understandings for dementia-related changes, developing a re-enablement programme and offering practical help. Ongoing flexible access to the community nurse, who understood Julie's emotional needs, was the key to managing her developing mood disorder (Chapters 3 and 10), and to minimising the risk of 'social pathology' and progressive disabilities for Darren. Darren maintained his walks and gardening pleasures until he died peacefully 16 months later in hospital, following a chest infection. Julie now befriends other carers, often helping with practical tasks such as taking them to the supermarket. She reports feeling more useful and less lonely. This case illustration describes how timely psychosocial interventions (such as cognitive, physical, social and pleasurable activity) that were delivered when needed and acceptable helped maintain psychosocial wellbeing or 'social health' (see Chapters 2, 6, 10 and 11). Of note is that one part of the dyad (the person with dementia) would not have accepted a post-diagnostic 'watchful waiting' or a monitoring brief, had it been part of the offer at the memory clinic five years previously; whist the other part (the 'carer') needed ongoing emotional support following knowledge that her husband had dementia.

Family and carer support
The move from being a family member to a carer is sometimes gradual but can be sudden. The pre-existing relationship may have been close, may have been positive and may have been long-standing. The opposite,

of course, can apply, and for most this is likely to be a grey area with ambivalence, uncertainty and a mixture of emotions. This means that psychosocial interventions for carers need to be as person-centred as for the person with dementia (Manthorpe and Samsi 2016). Other resources may also need to be considered – making use of strengths-based or community-asset approaches (IRIS 2014; Rahman and Swaffer 2018; SCIE 2011). These can help in problem solving, individual support and group psycho-educational workshops where carers follow up initial family conversations post-diagnosis. Components may include communication-skills training, targeting improvements of listening or conversation, and introduction to the principles of emotion-orientated communication, where anxieties may be validated to reduce episodes of disorientation (Chapter 11).

Across Europe there is growing interest in responding to the many cultures that are part of the dementia workforce and being more inclusive of people with dementia and carers from different backgrounds, such as religious, ethnic or national minorities (IRIS 2014; Nielsen *et al.* 2011). Many of the following chapters use examples from practice with migrants or people of minority cultures and backgrounds and the practitioners involved are also from diverse backgrounds. The final case of Davud and his wife Lejla is an example of such diversity; it also illustrates the need to listen to family carers who are often valuable sources of information about past lives and previous coping strategies.

Case Study 1.6 – **Davud and Lejla**

Davud's wife Lejla was concerned about his visual hallucinations. Davud often mistook his dressing gown, hung on his bedroom door, as a person standing in the bedroom. He was getting anxious about this and often begged the person to go away. Lejla was highly distressed about this, worrying that he might no longer recognise her or that the 'person' might reawaken her husband's war memories.

During a carers' group meeting (taking the form of a workshop) the nurse showed a functional diagram of the brain to explain how occipital lobe damage could be contributing to Davud's visual disturbances, which were often temporarily worse when he was over-stimulated, such as at night-time. During the workshop, Irena, the daughter of a man with vascular dementia, added how she and her father had, with support, reduced the frequency of such 'misperceptions'. Jeanne, another carer, reported that she had found the book *The Man Who Mistook His Wife for a Hat* (Sachs 1970), helpful in understanding similar difficulties in her mother.

Lejla felt more reassured that her husband's 'hallucinations' were associated with 'tricks of the brain' rather than the first step to his being unable to recognise her or the re-awakening of his war-time trauma; she had also shared such trauma, having lost many members of her family in post-war population relocations. The possibility of his traumatic experiences re-emerging was noted by the nurse and formed part of care-planning information given to care staff when this became more evident. Lejla's own feelings of loss but also her resilience were also acknowledged.

Conclusions

The psychosocial interventions described in this book illustrate the three components of a framework for psychosocial interventions in dementia. They target health promotion, ways to pre-empt negative reactions, and support for people with dementia and carers throughout the dementia trajectory. All aspects of this may counteract dementia-related 'learned helplessness' (Flannery 2002), which is a psychological state associated with mood disorder, when a person who is unable to control one situation incorrectly assumes that they are unable to exercise reasonable control in other situations as well. This can occur when a family carer is exhausted by broken nights and feels the pressure to keep cheerful and is also illustrated in Case Study 1.5 (Darren and Julie) where disengagement and potential factors associated with social pathology were present. Learned helplessness may arise from poor or rushed practice, such as getting someone dressed when they can manage some of this activity themselves, if slowly.

Psychosocial interventions in care homes to assist in reducing learned helplessness or disengagement can take many forms (Lawrence *et al.* 2012). Some of these are described in Chapters 12 to 16. There is a further dimension in the framework for reducing excess disability in dementia. This provides psychological treatment for people and their carers who are depressed or anxious (Livingston *et al.* 2013). Examples to alleviate mood problems for those in the home setting are seen in Chapters 3, 8, 10 and 11; and music or other activity-based programmes are helpful in care homes (Chapters 12 and 14).

As many chapters in this book note, delivering timely psychosocial interventions is not always straightforward. Engagement in intervention often depends on the attitudes, beliefs and aspirations of the person, their spouse or partner and their wider family or support systems. Where differing attitudes, beliefs and aspirations or tensions exist, psycho-educational family conferences (Chapter 10) may help, or separate practitioners may be required to meet the aspirations of the person with dementia and of the carer (Chapter 3). However, for most families, the programmes described here demonstrate that skilled practitioners can offer psychosocial interventions over the full dementia trajectory, including when people with dementia are at non-verbal or advanced stages of the condition (Chapters 15 and 16). The importance of the care setting's organisational culture must be acknowledged (Goodman *et al.* 2017), with managers, owners, supervisors and colleagues all impacting on proposed changes, and with interests, sometimes, in keeping things as they are.

Communication lies at the heart of all we do. It surrounds any and all psychosocial interventions, and yet aspects of communication may be overlooked. In dementia care practice, communication is often framed as a problem, notably with the person with dementia, whose symptoms may include some difficulties with expression or severe problems communicating and being understood. At times communication problems can arise between people with dementia and their family carers – as touched on in several chapters (see Chapters 3, 15 and 17).

This book itself is part of communication between researchers and practitioners and between researchers working in different national contexts, building on the well-established links of the INTERDEM network.[3] However, new elements of communication are needed in dementia-care practice. These extend to the need for legal literacy when advocating for people with dementia and to hearing the voices of dementia advocates. Services and professionals are increasingly being challenged by people with dementia, with a human rights approach (Bartlett *et al.* 2018; Cahill 2018) to counter discrimination, social exclusion and disengagement. Likewise, research increasingly needs to involve and engage people with dementia, and there is a growing evidence base of the impact of these communications (Gove *et al.* 2018). Dementia-care practice has to involve people affected by dementia in

---

3   www.interdem.org

making decisions about their own care, treatment and service design, and about the skills they expect to see offered to them by practitioners.

References

Age UK (2018) *Why Call It Care When Nobody Cares?* London: Age UK.

Ahmadi-Abhari, S., Guzman-Castillo, M., Bandosz, P., Shipley, M.J. *et al.* (2017) 'Temporal trend in dementia incidence since 2002 and projections for prevalence in England and Wales to 2040: Modelling study.' *British Medical Journal 358*, j2856.

Bartlett, R., Gjernes, T., Lotherington, A. and Obstefelder, A. (2018) 'Gender, citizenship and dementia care: A scoping review of studies to inform policy and future research.' *Health and Social Care in the Community 26*, 1, 14–26.

British Psychological Society (2018) *Psychological Dimensions of Dementia: Putting the Person at the Centre of Care.* Leicester: British Psychological Society. Accessed on 7/4/2019 at www.bps.org.uk/news-and-policy/psychological-dimensions-dementia

Cahill, S. (2018) *Dementia and Human Rights.* Bristol: Policy Press.

Campbell, S., Manthorpe, J., Samsi, K., Abley, C. *et al.* (2016) 'Living with uncertainty: Mapping the transition from pre-diagnosis to a diagnosis of dementia.' *Journal of Aging Studies 37*, 40–47.

Dröes, R.M., Chattat, R., Diaz, A., Gove, D. *et al.* and the INTERDEM Social Health Taskforce (2017) 'Social health and dementia: A European consensus on the operationalization of the concept and directions for research and practice.' *Aging and Mental Health 21*, 1, 4–17.

Evans, D., Price, K. and Meyer, J. (2016) 'Home alone with dementia.' *SAGE Open 6*, 3, 21582440166649. doi:10.1177/2158244016664954

Flannery, R. (2002) 'Treating learned helplessness in the elderly dementia patient: Preliminary inquiry.' *American Journal of Alzheimer's Disease and Other Dementias 17*, 6, 345–349.

Goodman, C., Sharpe, R., Russell, C., Meyer, J. *et al.* (2017) *Care Home Readiness: A Rapid Review and Consensus Workshops on How Organisational Context Affects Care Home Engagement with Health Care Innovation.* London: NHS England. Accessed on 7/4/2019 at https://doi.org/10.18745/pb.18200

Gove, D., Diaz-Ponce, A., Georges, J., Moniz-Cook, E. *et al.* (2018) 'Alzheimer Europe's position on involving people with dementia in research through PPI (patient and public involvement).' *Aging & Mental Health, 22*, 6, 723–729.

IRIS (2014) *Voices and Assets: Dementia in Black, Asian and Minority Ethnic Communities.* Stirling: Dementia Services Development Centre. Accessed on 7/4/2019 at http://dementia.stir.ac.uk/system/files/filedepot/24/02482_dsdc_iris_voices_and_assets_paper_09-1.pdf

Lawrence, V., Fossey, J., Ballard, C., Moniz-Cook, E. and Murray, J. (2012) 'Improving quality of life for people with dementia in care homes: Making psychosocial interventions work.' *British Journal of Psychiatry 201*, 344–351.

Livingston, G., Barber, J., Rapaport, P., Knapp, M. *et al.* (2013) 'Clinical effectiveness of a manual based coping strategy programme (START, STrAtegies for RelaTives) in promoting the mental health of carers of family members with dementia: Pragmatic randomised controlled trial.' *British Medical Journal 347*, f6276.

Livingston, G., Sommerlad A., Orgeta, V., Costafreda, S. *et al.* (2017) 'Dementia prevention, intervention, and care.' *Lancet 390*, 10113, 2673–2734.

Low, L.F., Swaffer, K., McGrath, M. and Brodaty, H. (2018) 'Do people with early stage dementia experience Prescribed Disengagement'? A systematic review of qualitative studies.' *International Psychogeriatrics 30*, 6, 807–831.

Maidment, I., Aston, L., Moutela, T., Fox, C. and Hilton, A. (2017) 'A qualitative study exploring medication management in people with dementia living in the community and the potential role of the community pharmacist.' *Health Expectations 20*, 5, 929–942.

Manthorpe, J., Hart, C., Watts, S., Fossey, J. *et al.* (2018) 'Practitioners' understanding of barriers to accessing specialist support by family carers of people with dementia in distress.' *International Journal of Care and Caring 2*, 1, 109–123.

Manthorpe, J. and Samsi, K. (2016) 'Person-centered dementia care: Current perspectives.' *Clinical Interventions in Aging 11*, 1733–1740.

Mitchell, W. (2018) *Somebody I Used to Know*. London: Bloomsbury.

Moniz-Cook, E.D., Manthorpe, J., Carr, I., Gibson, G. and Vernooij-Dassen, M. (2006) 'Facing the future: A qualitative study of older people referred to a memory clinic prior to assessment and diagnosis.' *Dementia 5*, 3, 375–395.

Nielsen, T., Vogel, A., Riepe, M., Mendonca, A. *et al.* (2011) 'Assessment of dementia in ethnic minority patients in Europe: A European Alzheimer's Disease Consortium survey.' *International Psychogeriatrics 23*, 1, 86–95.

Patterson, K., Clarke, C., Wolverson, E. and Moniz-Cook, E.D. (2018) 'Through the eyes of others – the social experiences of people with dementia: A systematic literature review and synthesis.' *International Psychogeriatrics 30*, 6 791–805

Poulos, C.J., Bayer, A., Beaupre, L., Clare, L. *et al.* (2017) 'A comprehensive approach to reablement in dementia.' *Alzheimer's and Dementia 3*, 3, 450–458.

Rahman, S. and Swaffer, K. (2018) 'Assets-based approaches and dementia-friendly communities.' *Dementia 17*, 2, 131–137.

Sachs, O. (1970) *The Man Who Mistook His Wife for a Hat*. New York: Simon and Schuster.

SCIE (2011) Windows of *Opportunity: Prevention and Early Intervention in Dementia*. London: Social Care Institute for Excellence. Accessed on 7/4/2019 at www.scie.org.uk/ publications/windowsofopportunity/localassets/assetbasedworking.asp

Sharma, S., Mueller, C., Stewart, R., Veronese, N. *et al.* (2018) 'Predictors of falls and fractures leading to hospitalization in people with dementia: A representative cohort study.' *Journal of the American Medical Directors Association 19*, 7, 607–612.

Surr, C.A., Gates, C., Irving, D., Oyebode, J. and Smith, S.J. (2017) 'Effective dementia education and training for the health and social care workforce: A systematic review of the literature.' *Review of Educational Research 87*, 5, 966–1002.

Sutin, A.R., Yannick S.R., Luchetti, M. and Terracciano, A. (2018) 'Loneliness and risk of dementia.' *Journals of Gerontology: Series B*, e-pub. doi:10.1093/geronb/gby112

Swaffer, K. (2015) 'Dementia and prescribed disengagement.' *Dementia 14*, 1, 3–6.

Takahashi, K., Tamura, J. and Tokoro, M. (1997) 'Patterns of social relationships and psychological well-being among the elderly.' *International Journal of Behavioral Development 21*, 3, 417–430.

Teri, L. and Truax, P. (1994) 'Assessment of depression in dementia patients: Associations of carer mood with depression ratings.' *Gerontologist 34*, 231–234.

Vernooij-Dassen, M. and Jeon, Y-H. (2016) 'Social health and dementia: The power of human capabilities.' *International Psychogeriatrics 28*, 5, 701–703.

Vernooij Dassen, M., Moniz-Cook, E. and Jeon, Y-H. (2018) 'Social health in dementia: Harnessing an applied research agenda.' *International Psychogeriatrics 30*, 6, 775–778.

Windle, G., Gregory, S., Howson-Griffiths, T., Newman, A., O'Brien, D. and Goulding, A. (2017) 'The impact of a visual arts program on quality of life, communication, and well-being of people living with dementia: A mixed-methods longitudinal investigation.' *International Psychogeriatrics 30*, 409–423.

PART 1

Preventing Disability: Post-Diagnostic Support

Early diagnosis of dementia has become the gateway for people to access post-diagnostic support. Practitioners can from the start help people living with dementia and their families to have as good a life as possible, by maintaining their health and wellbeing. This part of the book outlines ways in which practitioners can work with people and their families and friends, to make decisions about evidence-based support programmes that might suit them best, and what ongoing contact they might require through their journey with dementia. Each chapter outlines a key support programme from different countries across Europe.

Chapter 2

Choosing Psychosocial Interventions for People with Dementia and Their Families

PROTOCOLS FOR DECISION-MAKING

Esme Moniz-Cook and Chris Rewston

Introduction

Dementia remains a complex condition with variable impacts upon the person, their family and their interpersonal and social settings. Research is at an early stage of providing structured practical advice for practitioners on how to select psychosocial intervention(s) for a given person and their family carer. This may be due to the reliance of the current evidence base on randomised controlled studies, where statistical results of individually tailored support programmes may report effectiveness of an intervention for the 'average person', but rarely do these provide detail on who might not benefit, who might not wish to receive the intervention, or about the complexity of individual characteristics that have to be taken into account when making decisions about care (Butler *et al.* 2018). Thus practitioners often require other types of knowledge to make judgements about how to provide evidence-based care for specific individuals (Pearce, Raman and Turner 2015).

Rational decision-making refers to a structured reasoning process for making decisions about which interventions might suit a particular person at a given time. These standardised protocols integrate 'person-centred' aspects with psychiatric diagnostic approaches (Groenier *et al.* 2011; Mast 2012) or, in the absence of psychiatric diagnoses, they are described variously as 'care diagnoses' (Vermandere, Decloedt and De

Lepeleire 2012) and 'formulation-based approaches' (Baird *et al.* 2017; British Psychological Society 2011; Hughes 2016; Royal College of Psychiatrists 2013). In dementia services these formulaic 'algorithm-based' protocols are emerging to help practitioners make judgements about diagnoses (Lee, Weston and Hillier 2018), interventions for managing depression in people with dementia (see Chapter 14), behavioural problems (Kales, Gitlin and Lyketsos 2015; Kovach *et al.* 2012; Ryan *et al.* 2018; Teipel *et al.* 2017) and support for family carers (Marziali, McCleary and Streiner 2010; Pepin *et al.* 2013; Pini *et al.* 2017). Of note is that rational decision-making in dementia differs from other long-term conditions – it is influenced by personal rather than practical aspects, including questions of involvement of the person with dementia in decision-making (Fetherstonhaugh, Tarzia and Nay 2013), potential reliance on others for decision-making and strong emotions, which are time-consuming, especially at the exploration (assessment) phase (Wolfs *et al.* 2012).

The difficulties associated with dementia often occur within the context of each person's and their family's social environment (Bunn *et al.* 2012). Cognitive decline is only one factor in the person's adjustment. Other factors, such as the carer's past and current emotional wellbeing and other family characteristics may all influence the level of disability that emerges following diagnosis (Clare *et al.* 2012). This means that assessment for the delivery of any psychosocial intervention in dementia care should include the person and their family carer (if there is one), since these 'dyadic interventions' are more effective than pharmacological approaches (Laver *et al.* 2016). However, access to evidence-based effective psychosocial interventions is limited, since few have been translated into routine care (Clemson *et al.* 2018). Three examples of where this has occurred are: the 'Reducing disability in Alzheimer's Disease – RDAD' multicomponent intervention, conceived in Seattle in the USA in 1998, published as an effective intervention in 2003, now delivered by local care provider agencies (Teri *et al.* 2018); Mittleman's New York family caregiver counselling intervention, published in 1995, and tested in different contexts with varying degrees of success (see Chapter 10); and The Netherlands' community occupational therapy intervention published in 2006 (Graff *et al.* 2006), applied in routine practice and tested in other European countries with varying success (Dopp *et al.* 2015; Graff 2015; Pozzi *et al.* 2018; Voigt-Radloff *et al.* 2011; Wenbourn *et al.* 2016).

The early memory clinic psychosocial intervention studies from Hull, in England (undertaken late 1990s–2000), were delivered following communication of a dementia diagnosis, where care was taken to discuss the meaning of the diagnosis with people and as many of their family members as possible. This aimed to neutralise potential effects of stigma at the time of diagnosis or 'prescribed disengagement' (see Chapter 1). In the first study (Moniz-Cook *et al.* 1998) a three-month in-home individualised psychosocial intervention, involving the family in cognitive rehabilitation (see Chapter 7) was used. Initially at six-month follow-up, carers were more distressed compared with the 'treatment-as-usual' group; but by 18 months, when compared 'treatment-as-usual', there was a significant positive effect on carer mood and on memory in people with dementia and more people with dementia were still living at home. In the second study (Moniz-Cook *et al.* 2001) behavioural activation (pleasurable activity), health promotion and carer counselling components were added to cognitive rehabilitation. This time there were slightly increased levels of carer stress at six months, compared with 'treatment-as-usual', but by 12 months carers reported significantly less burden with improved coping and fewer problems; people with dementia were less depressed and more of them were being cared for at home.

This chapter will outline a protocol that grew out of these studies, as a clinical tool at diagnosis in a memory clinic, which facilitated judgements about psychosocial care.

Targeting psychosocial interventions

The key to successful psychosocial interventions is that they are individualised to the person and carer, based on a psychosocial disability risk appraisal of the person–carer dyad; and that professional support is available and responsive to their changing needs. This type of tailored approach to offering support is important, since any intervention has to be both meaningful and relevant to the person and/or the family. Using diagnostic or other criteria such as early, moderate and advanced dementia or hierarchical stepped-care approaches at this important time of adjustment to a dementia diagnosis runs the risk of undermining engagement with some families by failing to address their subtle and often nuanced needs when first seeking help (Vermandere *et al.* 2012). People seek help at very different times and for different reasons.

Therefore, the entry point for people seeking psychosocial assistance is personal to their current, potentially very varied, circumstances. A 'one-size-fits-all' or 'stepped-care approach' to psychosocial interventions without a good appreciation of people and their family contexts can result in poor uptake, refusal to accept potentially helpful interventions (Rogers *et al.* 2014) or indeed in a loss of faith in services that could be of help currently or in the future. The six case illustrations outlined in Chapter 1 demonstrate the variety of factors that were taken into account to meet the needs of the person with dementia and their carer.

The aim of a psychosocial assessment at the time of a dementia diagnosis is to map the potential risks of psychosocial disability that reduces wellbeing in people and family carers and then to consider relevant opportunities for mental, physical and occupational activities or for social support to prevent or reduce these risks. Social isolation, disengagement and loss of personal identity are just some of the commonly reported risks for people with dementia, while distress and burnout are risks for carers (Bunn *et al.* 2012). Not all people and family carers have the same risk profiles (Fulmer *et al.* 2005); some may be more vulnerable than others depending on their strengths and assets, their personality, relationships, physical and emotional health, and their social and financial circumstances; some may accept help, whilst other may be prone to rejecting this (see Case Study 2.2 – Mr Walters[1]); some types of interventions may be more relevant for some but not others; and some families may require sustained oversight from skilled professionals (described here as 'case management'), whilst others may only require a 'lighter-touch approach' from professionals. There may also be different needs: the person may feel self-conscious about word-finding problems and without encouragement can actively disengage from social situations (Donkers *et al.* 2018); or a carer may become excessively anxious about their perceived 'loss of their relative' (Feast *et al.* 2016), or the person and the carer may have differing aspirations following diagnosis (Moon *et al.* 2017), or the balance of the relationship between the person and carer may shift (Conway *et al.* 2018).

---

1   A pseudonym, as are all names in case studies in this chapter.

The Hull Memory Clinic Decision Tree

The Hull Memory Clinic Decision Tree is rational means of assisting practitioners to engage collaboratively with people with dementia and their families in offering support to adjust to a dementia diagnosis and maintain engagement in everyday life. This person–carer psychosocial disability risk appraisal involves gathering and examining information about potential vulnerabilities (see Clare *et al.* 2012), and strengths (such as interests, close social relationships and cultural network resources), which may balance out some of these vulnerabilities. These are then used to inform interventions that might suit the person and their family carer at a given time.

Good assessment data and experienced clinical judgement help to identify the factors for both the carer and the person with dementia that are markers to potential poorer outcomes following a dementia diagnosis. Central to making use of this data is the process of 'case formulation'. Three clinically relevant factors are important in the tailoring of interventions offered to newly diagnosed people with a dementia, and the families:

- *Pre-existing vulnerabilities in the person with dementia and/or the carer.* These could be historical mood disorder(s), coping styles, social isolation or family conflict. This is used to make a judgement on whether there is a high or low 'vulnerability risk' of psychosocial disability.

- *The level of current distress of the person with dementia.* For example, current mood disorder, agitation or risk of self-harm would be considered 'high' need.

- *A carer's current emotional and physical health and levels of distress/burden.* These include changes in the balance of the relationship – a carer might struggle with tasks that were the responsibility of their spouse; their adult children may be making demands; or a key adult-child carer may have other demands in addition to supporting their parent.

Taking these three factors into account offers the opportunity to systematically identify 'profiles of need' that may be linked to the most efficacious and appropriate evidence-based psychosocial treatments. Figure 2.1 outlines this structured process.

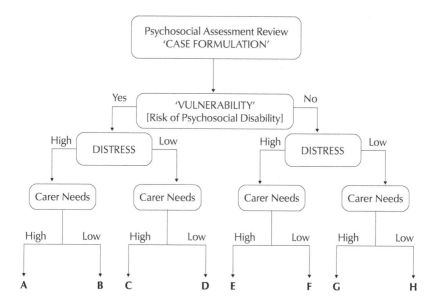

FAMILY 'NEED': PROFILES FOR PSYCHOSOCIAL INTERVENTION

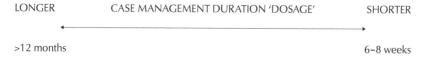

Figure 2.1: The Hull Memory Clinic Decision Tree

Using the process illustrated in Figure 2.1 over several years we identified eight psychosocial 'profiles of need' (listed as A–H), for estimating the degree of case management and approaches to psychosocial interventions. Each is designed to offer families a 'menu' of suitable initial post-diagnostic support for minimising potential risks in adjusting to the dementia diagnosis. The interventions identified (Table 2.1) are just indicative of the type of relevant support. Key to tailoring interventions is the practitioner's detailed local knowledge about what is available; and perhaps, more relevant, a good understanding of what meaningful activities the person and family are (or were) engaged in, that can be maintained or reinstated if possible (see also Chapter 1 case illustrations, Jenny and Darren). Often a key task for the practitioner is to discuss with the person and family how they might manage the obstacles to maintaining mental, physical and meaningful social activities and participate in family life and their local communities.

The degree of case management involvement can differ according to the needs identified in the decision process. For example, someone assessed as having no past or current vulnerabilities may be offered support within menu 'H' and short-term case management. Alternatively, in the cases presenting with high vulnerability where the person and carer are at increased risk of psychosocial disabilities, menu 'A' and longer-term case management would be relevant. Ongoing case-management review would also be informed by the practitioner's evaluation of family stability as they engage with psychosocial intervention. Table 2.1 outlines some of the indicative interventions that can be explored with the person and family.

Table 2.1: Timely post-diagnostic psychosocial
intervention: Profile-based menus for support

Profile	Menus of post-diagnostic psychosocial interventions
A	**Dyad-focused:** High risk of psychosocial disability for both person and carer. Key to intervention is the initial therapeutic strategy to engage the person and carer, drawing on family and social support strengths where they exist. Interventions include: individualised psycho-education, emotional support and regular contact with a therapist (Chapters 3, 8 and 10), the community occupational therapy intervention for people with dementia and carers (COTiD),[1] cognitive reframing,[2] management strategies and emotional support for the carer.[4] Group based interventions (Chapter 5, 11), social prescribing[6] activity opportunities (Chapter 6) and peer support (Chapter 4) can be considered later, with help to engage from the case manager. Monitoring unmet mental and physical health needs in the dyad is an important target for case management. **Post-diagnosis case-management duration: Long**
B	**Dyad-focused:** High risk of psychosocial disability in the person. This profile is similar to Profile A for the range of suitable psychosocial interventions for the person, but is of less risk of carer psychosocial disability. With encouragement, the carer may actively learn skills and strategies,[3,4] and facilitate relevant psychosocial interventions (see Chapters 4–7 and 9, individual cognitive stimulation therapy iCST[6] or life story work[7]). The focus is on the carer's support of their relative with reducing case management intensity over 12 months. Monitoring for unmet need(s) in both person and carer is an important target for the case manager reviews. **Post-diagnosis case-management duration: Long**

C	**Carer-focused:** High risk of carer psychosocial disability.
	Key to initial psychosocial intervention an active therapeutic strategy to engage the carer and their family and social supports; whilst not ignoring their person with dementia. Initial individual 'couples' support is indicated to foster trust and the carer's adjustment to changed circumstances. Intervention components alongside this include those outlined in Chapters 3, 4, 5, 9, 10 and 11; strategies to manage day-to-day problems,[1,3,4] social support,[5] followed by couples group approaches such as meeting places (see Chapter 4). Monitoring unmet need in the carer is an important target for case management.
	Post-diagnosis case-management duration: Medium
D	**Dyad-focused:** High risk of psychosocial disability for both person and carer.
	This profile reflects reluctance by the person to accept timely support, often when there are likely to be difficulties with adjustment and/or acceptance of dementia. The therapeutic strategy is one of 'assertive engagement', where the case manager maintains a 'respectful distance' ('watchful waiting') using telephone or 'pop-in' contact with the family, aimed at monitoring family stability and offering timely support.
	Post-diagnosis case-management duration: Long-Medium
E	**Carer-focused:** High risk of carer psychosocial disability.
	This profile is similar to Profile C, for approach and interventions for the carer.
	Key to initial psychosocial intervention an active therapeutic strategy to engage the carer and their family and social supports. There is less risk of disability for the person with dementia if adequate support is offered to the carer.
	Monitoring unmet need in the carer is an important target for case management.
	Post-diagnosis case-management duration: Long-Medium
F	**Dyad-focused:** High risk of psychosocial disability in the person.
	This profile is similar to Profile B: individualised/group psychological therapy (see Chapter 8) if the person will accept this; the carer may actively learn skills and strategies,[3,4] and facilitate relevant psychosocial interventions (see Chapters 4 –7 and 9, individual cognitive stimulation therapy iCST,[6] life story work[7]) and uptake of social prescribing opportunities.[5] This may also involve individually formulated support [3] for dementia-related distressing symptoms.[4] Following stability within the family, monitoring for unmet need(s) in both person and carer is an important target for case management.
	Post-diagnosis case-management duration: Long-Medium

cont.

TIMELY PSYCHOSOCIAL INTERVENTIONS IN DEMENTIA CARE

G	**Carer-focused:** High risk of carer psychosocial disability.
	Individual[2,4] and/or group counselling (Chapters 3,10 and 11) for the carer. This may also involve individually formulated support for dementia-related distressing symptoms.[4] Interventions for the person with dementia or the dyad (both person and carer) as outlined in Profile H, including encouraging others in the family or wider social network to support the dyad. Following a stable package of support, monitoring carer unmet need is an important target for case management.
	Post-diagnosis case management duration: Short-Medium
H	**Dyad-focused:** Psycho-education – support required to adjust to diagnosis.
	Facilitating a healthy lifestyle aimed at empowering people and carers to maintain their mental, physical, occupational and their usual enjoyable social activities (see Chapters 3 and 6). People with dementia who are currently socially isolated or enjoy meeting new people could be offered the seven-week group cognitive stimulation therapy (see Chapter 5), whilst more private people may prefer individualised cognitive rehabilitation (see Chapter 7). Others may simply require support to engage (or re-engage) with socialising in their local communities. Some may benefit from signposting to local supportive agencies (e.g. Dementia Cafés – Chapter 4).
	Post-diagnosis case-management duration: Short

Key

Interventions: [1] Graff 2015; [2] Vernooij-Dassen *et al.* 2011; [3] Moniz-Cook *et al.* 2012; [4] Livingston *et al.* 2013; [5] Thomson, Camic and Chatterjee 2015; [6] Orrell *et al.* 2017; [7] Kaiser and Eley 2016

Case management: Longer-term = 12 months post-diagnosis; with 6-month review thereafter (these may be reduced dependent on family stability). Medium term = > 6 months < 12 months) post-diagnosis; 6-month review or less, or telephone review dependent family stability. Short term = 12–20 weeks post-diagnosis; 6 (telephone) to 12-month review depending on family efficacy and stability.

Case studies: Description of profiles

Profile A

This profile reflects people with dementia and carers known to have current and past vulnerabilities through their poor coping with adverse events. Many will have received previous mental health services for mood problems before their dementia symptoms emerged. However, the absence of mental health problems may not necessarily exclude being categorised in this profile, since a history of poor coping responses – such as substance misuse, avoidance coping styles, difficulties in maintain close relationships through life, suicidal thinking – may affect the person. This profile can also include people with young-onset dementia – some may be at work with financially dependent families, requiring paced and longer-term post-diagnostic support and case-management planning as their route to diagnosis and associated uncertainties could require significant emotional support before they adjust to living life with the condition. The clinician's judgement is obviously vital here.

Case Study 2.1 – **Mrs Bilton**

Mrs Bilton was referred to the memory clinic following concerns about her increasing forgetfulness, of three years duration. Her husband had been reluctant to seek help since his wife, who had suffered several episodes of depression throughout her life, had often threatened to 'end it all' should she have to go into a care home. Therefore he had not encouraged her to seek support and actively discouraged his two daughters from voicing their concerns. This had resulted in reduced contact and support from them. Mrs Bilton managed most of her own personal care and housework, but with increasing assistance from her husband.

Cognitive screening showed significant deficits in orientation, encoding and recall of new information, and poor visual planning. Mrs Bilton's mood was also problematic, with high levels of anxious worrying, feelings of panic and pessimism about the future. Her husband had clinically significant levels of anxiety, and high scores on instruments measuring carer stress and burden. These were linked to his feelings of responsibility in keeping his wife safe.

This profile informed the support offered at the 'diagnostic feedback' meeting, where Mr and Mrs Bilton attended with one of their daughters. It recognised both current and past vulnerabilities to receiving a diagnosis, with individual and family-based psycho-education as the key initial psychosocial intervention. Empathic understanding of Mrs Bilton's fears and her assumptions around dementia enabled practitioners to discuss with her and her family the range of opportunities that they could engage in, to minimise disability and manage fear. An individualised couples' intervention, rather that group-based support, focused on encouragement to engage in enjoyable social activities, until mood in both parts of the dyad had improved. Phasing into community groups to meet others in the same situation either as a couple (see Chapter 4) or on their own (see Chapters 5, 10 and 11) could be a later option for psychosocial support. Ongoing specialist case management is an important aspect of support for this profile.

Profile D

This profile reflects people who are identified as being vulnerable to adjustment or of not accepting the dementia diagnosis. There is little current expression of distress in either the person or the family carer. This may be due to the current environment being sufficiently structured to minimise distress or it may reflect a reluctance to acknowledge the emerging memory problems.

Case Study 2.2 – **Mr Walters**

Mr Walters (aged 71) was encouraged to seek help by his daughter Carol. Her concerns centred on her father becoming increasingly dependent upon reminders about conversations they had had and increasing episodes of him losing his belongings around the home. Although Mr Walters did not believe his memory was problematic, he agreed to his family doctor's suggestion to visit the memory clinic. Mr Walters attended the clinic with his wife.

The assessment found that he was suffering some significant problems in planning and retaining new information, and a diagnosis of Alzheimer's disease was indicated. No obvious mood difficulties were noted, and Mr Walters was keen to emphasise that everything was 'alright'. His medical notes confirmed that Mr Walter's had not made much use of health services in the past and there were no current active medical conditions, or history of mental health problems. Mr Walters was apparently a 'private, autonomous man' who did not like others 'interfering in his affairs'. It emerged that Mr Walters had left his job as a gardener at the age of 51 due to back pain and he had then held a number of jobs prior to his retirement at 65. He has found it difficult to get along with people and, according to his wife, he was a worrier by nature and was not comfortable with socialising. Mrs Walters emphasised her concern that services would 'upset the applecart' by undermining their privacy. Mr Walters declined a home assessment of his activities in daily living, and any other psychosocial support, but was willing to accept cholinesterase inhibitor drug treatment. The family's vulnerability to psychosocial disability was seen as high – although there were current problems the risk of this couple's further needs becoming 'hidden' until it was too late to prevent distress and disability was noted and a profile of D was assigned to their care plan.

The emphasis for this profile is on ensuring contact is available at times when they feel ready to engage whilst 'keeping respectful distance'. Proposals at post-diagnostic feedback were to keep in telephone contact with them and their daughter, aimed at building trust and family stability through ensuring that one person would be their point of contact either by telephone or inviting them to ring or 'drop in' to the clinic. This was acceptable to the family and allowed them to maintain their autonomy but also access information, advice and support, which became important to meeting their needs later in the dementia trajectory.

Profile H

Many people approach services with a positive philosophy towards memory decline and dementia. Where people have no identified past or current emotional vulnerabilities the profile of H is assigned. In this profile empowering the individual is the aim, and case management and the interventions offered seek to maintain independence and enable families to manage the condition without memory services being too intrusive.

Case Study 2.3 – **Mr Milne**

Mr Milne had noticed he was becoming more forgetful over the last year. His wife shared his concerns and described episodes where he would repeatedly need reminders about appointments or people's names. Both had discussed this and agreed to see the GP together.

At the memory clinic Mr Milne said he wanted a diagnosis so that he could understand what was happening and what he could do about it. Mrs Milne stated that they had been through many things together and would do this if dementia was found; neither had significant levels of anxiety or depression. There were no previous problems with mood or coping styles. Mr Milne was socially active, enjoying helping at his local church and going out with friends. His family regularly visited and Mr Milne stressed that as long as he and his wife were able to live independently then they would be fine. A diagnosis of Alzheimer's disease was confirmed and the profile H decided upon.

At the feedback appointment both Mr and Mrs Milne were offered interventions to encourage their continued independence. They were provided with education and information materials about the condition and what NHS-recommended treatments were available, such as cognitive stimulation and medication. In addition, they were given details of local activities for people living with memory difficulties. Mr and Mrs Milne were confident that they would enjoy these events and would make contact if they had difficulty finding them.

Profiles in a memory clinic

Table 2.2 shows the percentage distribution of psychosocial profiles formulated within the Hull Memory Clinic over a six-month period.

Table 2.2: Profile distribution of formulated cases over six months ($N = 417$)

Profile code	A	B	C	D	E	F	G	H
Percentage	3	4	3	6	7	9	22	46

The majority of cases (Profiles H and G) have relatively low complexity of need since they have little no complicating historical or current risk factors. Some carers (those in Profile G) required more support than others, for example, with the management of distressing dementia-related symptoms that can go unrecognised in the absence of a good assessment. Taken together, most (68%) of the 417 families did not require intensive case management over the following year. However, practitioners remained aware of the potentially changing needs within families and requirements for timely follow-up. Profiles A–D are considered as having greater care needs across the eight profiles. Over the 12 months, these four profiles were identified in 16 per cent of cases. They are typically characterised by care challenges either in isolation or in combination with engagement with post-diagnostic offers of support, problematic coping behaviour, and distressed responses to a diagnosis of dementia. The three cases in Profile A had the highest care complexity, due to both problematic historical and current coping responses. These required protracted specialist support for the person and their families but they were a minority.

The distributions outlined in Table 2.2 may not be an accurate representation of the spread of psychosocial need within the wider population; there may be a larger number of people and carers affected by dementia who are reluctant to actively engage with either their family doctor and/or specialist services to seek support. As health services begin to develop primary carer screening for dementia identification, we may see an increase in people with greater immediate care needs who may have been missed in the past. For example, a recent study in England noted people with mild dementia at home had higher levels of distressing dementia symptoms than people with dementia living in care homes (Moniz-Cook *et al.* 2017), and that the needs of family carers, even when referred to specialist services by their family doctor, could go unrecognised (British Psychological Society 2018; Manthorpe *et al.* 2018).

Conclusions

When designing psychosocial interventions and support, we have combined knowledge of family-based risk profiling (Fulmer *et al.* 2005), systemic theory as applied to dementia (Gonçalves-Pereira, Marques and Grácio 2017; Koehly 2017; Peisah 2006) and empirical evidence, to demonstrate the importance of evaluation of the family system at the start of a dementia diagnosis. The interventions outlined within these profiles are not 'prescriptions' or 'pills'. Developing relevant profile-based care plans relies on a good family assessment (see Moniz-Cook 2008, pp.427–428). Prior to use of our Decision Tree for planning proactive care, consideration of the basic premises and intervention approaches outlined in Chapter 1 is required. These should also include the much neglected group of self-care interventions that are specifically targeted at the family carer (Koehly 2017; Oliveira, Sousa and Orrell 2019) or the dyad. Protocols for recognising the wide-ranging need in dementia care are emerging (e.g. see Halek, Holle and Bartholomeyczik 2017; Kales *et al.* 2015; Kovach *et al.* 2012; Moniz-Cook *et al.* 2017; Ryan *et al.* 2018; Teipel *et al.* 2017; see also Chapter 14). These offer opportunity for practitioners in targeting their support to meet the sometimes 'hidden' needs of families (Manthorpe *et al.* 2018) and people with dementia living in care homes.

References

Baird, J., Hyslop, A., Macfie, M., Stocks, R. and Van der Kleij, T. (2017) 'Clinical formulation: Where it came from, what it is and why it matters.' *BJPsych Advances 23*, 2, 95–103.

British Psychological Society (2011) *Good Practice Guidelines on the Use of Psychological Formulation.* Accessed on 3/4/2019 at www.sisdca.it/public/pdf/DCP-Guidelines-for-Formulation-2011.pdf

British Psychological Society (2018) *Evidence briefing: 'Behaviour that challenges' in dementia.* Accessed on 2/4/2019 at www.bps.org.uk/sites/bps.org.uk/files/Policy/Policy%20-%20Files/Evidence%20briefing%20-%20behaviour%20that%20challenges%20in%20dementia.pdf

Bunn, F., Goodman, C., Sworn, K., Bryne, C. *et al.* (2012) 'Psychosocial factors that shape patient and carer experiences of dementia diagnosis and treatment: A systemic review of qualitative studies.' *PloS Med 9*, 10, e1001331.

Butler, C.C., Connor, J.T., Lewis, J.T., Broglio, K. *et al.* (2018) 'Answering patient-centred questions efficiently: Response-adaptive platform trials in primary care.' *British Journal of General Practice 68*, 671, 294–295.

Clare, L., Nelis, S.M., Martyr, A., Roberts, J. *et al.* (2012) 'The influence of psychological, social and contextual factors on the expression and measurement of awareness in early-stage dementia: Testing a biopsychosocial model.' *International Journal of Geriatric Psychiatry 27*, 167–177.

Clemson, L., Laver, K., Jeon, Y.H., Comans, T.A. *et al.* (2018) 'Implementation of an evidence-based intervention to improve the wellbeing of people with dementia and their carers: Study protocol for 'Care of People with dementia in their Environments (COPE)' in the Australian context.' *BMC Geriatrics, 18*, 108.

Conway, E., Watson, B., Tatangelo, G. and McCabe, M. (2018) 'Is it all bleak? A systematic review of factors contributing to relationship change in dementia.' *International Psychogeriatrics 30*, 11, 1619–1637.

Donkers, H.W., Vernooij-Dassen, M.J., van der Veen, D., van der Sanden, M.W.G. and Graff, M.J.L. (2018) 'Social participation perspectives of people with cognitive problems and their care-givers: A descriptive qualitative study.' *Ageing and Society*, 1–27.

Döpp, C.M., Graff, M.J., Teerenstra, S., Olde Rikkert, M.G. *et al.* (2015) 'Effectiveness of a training package for implementing a community-based occupational therapy program in dementia: A cluster randomized controlled trial.' *Clinical Rehabilitation 29*, 10, 974–986.

Feast, A., Orrell, M., Charlesworth, G., Melunsky, N., Poland, F. and Moniz-Cook, E. (2016) 'Behavioural and Psychological Symptoms in Dementia (BPSD) and the challenges for family carers: A systematic review.' *British Journal of Psychiatry 208*, 5, 429–434.

Fetherstonhaugh, D., Tarzia, L. and Nay, R. (2013) 'Being central to decision making means I am still here! The essence of decision making for people with dementia.' *Journal of Aging Studies 27*, 143–150.

Fulmer, T., Paveza, G., Vande Weerd, C., Fairchild, S. *et al.* (2005) 'Dyadic vulnerability and risk profiling.' *The Gerontologist, 45*, 4, 525–534.

Gonçalves-Pereira, M., Marques, M.J. and Grácio, J. (2017) 'Family Issues in Behavioral and Psychological Symptoms of Dementia: Unraveling Circular Pathways?' In A. Verdelho and M. Gonçalves-Pereira (eds) *Neuropsychiatric Symptoms in Cognitive Impairment and Dementia* (pp.331–348). New York: Springer.

Graff, M. (2015) 'Teaching and Supporting Clients with Dementia and Their Caregivers in Daily Functioning.' In I. Söderback (ed.) *International Handbook of Occupational Therapy Interventions* (pp.433–449). Cham, Switzerland: Springer International.

Graff, M J., Vernooij-Dassen, M.J, Thijssen, M., Dekker, J., Hoefnagels, W.H. and Rikkert, M.G. (2006) 'Community based occupational therapy for patients with dementia and their care givers: Randomised controlled trial.' *British Medical Journal 333*, 1196.

Groenier, M., Beerthuis, V., Pieters, J.M., Witteman, C. and Swinkels, J. (2011) 'Psychologists' diagnostic processes during a diagnostic interview.' *Psychology 2*, 917–924.

Halek, M., Holle, D. and Bartholomeyczik, S. (2017) 'Development and evaluation of the content validity, practicability and feasibility of the Innovative dementia-oriented Assessment system for challenging behaviour in residents with dementia.' *BMC Health Service Research 17*, 1, 554.

Hughes, P.M. (2016) 'Psychiatrists' use of formulation: Commentary on psychiatrists' understanding and use of psychological formulation.' *BJPsych Bulletin 40*, 4, 217–219.

Kaiser, P. and Eley, R. (2016) *Life Story Work with People with Dementia: Ordinary Lives Extraordinary People*. London: Jessica Kingsley Publishers.

Kales, H.C., Gitlin, L.N. and Lyketsos, C.J. (2015) 'Assessment and management of behavioural and psychological symptoms of dementia.' *British Medical Journal 350*, h369.

Koehly, L.M., (2017) 'It's interpersonal: Family relationships, genetic risk, and caregiving.' *The Gerontologist 57*, 1, 32–39.

Kovach, C.R., Simpson, M.R., Joossee, L., Logan, B.R. *et al.* (2012) 'Comparison of the effectiveness of two protocols for treating nursing home residents with advanced dementia.' *Research in Gerontological Nursing 5*, 4, 251–263.

Laver, K., Dyer, S., Whitehead, C., Clemson, L. and Crotty, M. (2016) 'Interventions to delay functional decline in people with dementia: A systematic review of systematic reviews.' *British Medical Journal Open 6*, 4, e010767.

Lee, L., Weston, W.W. and Hillier, L.M. (2018) 'Education to improve dementia care: Impact of a structured clinical reasoning approach.' *Family Medicine 50*, 3 195–203.

Livingston, G., Barber, J., Rapaport, P., Knapp, M. *et al.* (2013) 'Clinical effectiveness of a manual based coping strategy programme (START, STrAtegies for RelaTives) in promoting the mental health of carers of family members with dementia: Pragmatic randomised controlled trial.' *British Medical Journal 347*, f6276.

Manthorpe, J., Hart, C., Watts, S., Fossey, J. *et al.* (2018) 'Practitioners' understanding of barriers to accessing specialist support by family carers of people with dementia in distress.' *International Journal of Care and Caring 2*, 1, 109–123.

Marziali, E., McCleary, L. and Streiner, D.L. (2010) 'Evaluation of an assessment battery for estimating dementia caregiver needs for health and social carer services.' *American Journal of Alzheimer's Disease and Other Dementias 25*, 5, 446–454.

Mast, B.T. (2012) 'Methods for assessing the person with Alzheimer's disease: Integrating-person centred and diagnostic approaches to assessment.' *Clinical Gerontologist 35*, 360–375.

Moniz-Cook, E.D. (2008) 'Assessment and Psychosocial Intervention for Older People with Suspected Dementia: A Memory Clinic Perspective.' In K. Laidlaw and B. Knight (eds) *Handbook of Emotional Disorders in Late Life: Assessment and Treatment* (pp.421–451). Oxford: Oxford University Press.

Moniz-Cook, E., Gibson, G., Win, T., Agar, S. and Wang, M. (1998) 'A preliminary study of the effects of early intervention with people with dementia and their families in a memory clinic.' *Aging and Mental Health 2*, 166–175.

Moniz-Cook, E., Hart, C., Woods, B., Whitaker, C. *et al.* (2017) *Challenge Demcare: Management of Challenging Behaviour in Dementia at Home and in Care Homes*. Southampton: NIHR.

Moniz-Cook, E.D., Swift, K., James, I., Malouf, R., De Vugt, M. and Verhey, F. (2012) *Functional analysis-based interventions for challenging behaviour in dementia (review)*. The Cochrane Library, Issue 2.

Moniz-Cook, E., Wang, M., Campion, P., Gardiner, E. *et al.* (2001) 'Early psychosocial intervention through a memory: A randomised controlled trial.' *Gerontology 47*, 526.

Moon, H., Townsend, A.L., Whitlatch, C.J. and Dilworth-Anderson, P. (2017) Quality of life for dementia caregiving dyads: Effects of incongruent perceptions of everyday care and values.' *The Gerontologist 57*, 4, 657–666.

Oliveira, D., Sousa, L. and Orrell, M. (2019) 'Improving health-promoting self-care in family carers of people with dementia: A review of interventions.' *Clinical Interventions in Aging 14*, 515–523.

Orrell, M., Yates, L., Leung, P., Hoare, Z. *et al.* (2017) 'The impact of individual cognitive stimulation therapy (iCST) on cognition, quality of life, caregiver health, and family relationships in dementia: A randomized controlled trial.' *PloS Medicine 14*, 3, e1002269.

Pearce, W., Raman, S. and Turner, A. (2015) 'Randomised trials in context: Practical problems and social aspects of evidence-based medicine and policy.' *Trials 16*, 394.

Peisah, C. (2006) 'Practical application of family and systems theory in old age psychiatry: Three case reports.' *International Psychogeriatrics 18*, 2, 345–353.

Pepin, R., Williams, A.A., Anderson, L.N. and Qualls, S.H. (2013) 'A preliminary typology of caregivers and effects on service utilization of caregiver counselling.' *Aging & Mental Health 17*, 4, 495–507.

Pini, S., Ingleson, E., Megson, M., Clare, L., Wright, P. and Oyebode, R.J. (2017) 'A needs-led framework for understanding the impact of caring for a family member with dementia.' *The Gerontologist 58*, 2, e68–e77.

Pozzi, C., Lamzoni, A., Lucchi, E., Bergamini, L. *et al.* (2018) 'A pilot study of community-based occupational therapy for persons with dementia (COTID-IT) and their caregivers: Evidence for application in Italy.' [Epub ahead of print.] *Aging Clinical and Experimental Research.* doi:10.1007/s40520-018-1078-7

Rogers, A., Harris, T., Victor, C., Woodcock, A. *et al.* (2014) 'Which older people decline participation in a primary care trial of physical activity and why: Insights from a mixed methods approach.' *BMC Geriatrics 14*, 46.

Royal College of Psychiatrists (2013) *A Competency Based Curriculum for Specialist Core Training in Psychiatry*, CT1–CT3: pp.44–45. London: Royal College of Psychiatrists.

Ryan, N. P., Scott, L., McPhee, M. Mathers, S. *et al.* (2018) 'Evaluating the utility of a structured clinical protocol for reducing the impact of behavioural and psychological symptoms of dementia in progressive neurological diseases: A pilot study'. *Behavioural Neurology* Article ID 5420531.

Teipel, S., Heine, C., Hein, A., Krüger, F. *et al.* (2017) 'Multidimensional assessment of challenging behaviors in advanced stages of dementia in nursing homes: The insideDEM framework.' *Alzheimer's & Dementia: Diagnosis, Assessment & Disease Monitoring 8*, 36–44.

Teri, L., Logsdon, R.G., McCurry, S.M., Pike, K.C. and McGough, E.L. (2018) 'Translating an evidence-based multicomponent intervention for older adults with dementia and caregivers.' [Epub ahead of print.] *The Gerontologist.* doi:10.1093/geront/gny122

Thomson, L.J., Camic, P.M. and Chatterjee, H.J. (2015) *Social Prescribing: A Review Of Community Referral Schemes.* London: University College London.

Vermandere, M., Decloedt, P. and De Lepeleire, J. (2012) 'Care diagnosis for demented patients living at home: A new concept?' *Gerontology Geriatrics 43*, 26–33.

Vernooij-Dassen, M., Draskovic, I., McCleery, J. and Downs, M. (2011) 'Cognitive reframing for carers of people with dementia.' *Cochrane Database of Systematic Reviews*, Issue 11, Art. no. CD005318. doi:10.1002/14651858.CD005318.pub2

Voigt-Radloff, S., Graff, M., Leonhart, R., Hüll, M., Rikkert, M.O. and Vernooij-Dassen, M. (2011) 'Why did an effective Dutch complex psycho-social intervention for people with dementia not work in the German healthcare context? Lessons learnt from a process evaluation alongside a multicentre RCT.' *British Medical Journal Open 1*, e000094. doi:10.1136/bmjopen-2011-000094

Wenborn, J., Hynes, S., Moniz-Cook, E., Mountain, G. *et al.* (2016) 'Community occupational therapy for people with dementia and family carers (COTiD-UK) versus treatment as usual (Valuing Active Life in Dementia [VALID] programme): Study protocol for a randomised controlled trial.' *Trials 17*, 65.

Wolfs, C.A.G., de Vugt, M.E., Verkaaik, M., Haufe, M. *et al.* (2012) 'Rational decision-making about treatment and care in dementia: A contradiction in terms?' *Patient Education Counseling 87*,1, 43–48.

Related reading

Gonçalves-Pereira, M. (2017) 'Toward a Family-Sensitive Practice in Dementia.' In A. Verdelho and M. Gonçalves-Pereira (eds) *Neuropsychiatric Symptoms in Cognitive impairment and Dementia* (pp.349–368). New York: Springer. Social prescribing: www.kingsfund.org.uk/publications/social-prescribing

Evidence briefing (2015) University of York: www.york.ac.uk/media/crd/Ev%20briefing_social_prescribing.pdf

Chapter 3

Counselling People with Dementia and Their Families at Home

THE DAISY PROGRAMME

Ane Eckermann and Gunhild Waldemar

Introduction

Counselling and psychosocial interventions involving family carers of people with dementia can have a significant positive effect on people with dementia or, more commonly, their family carers (Brodaty *et al.* 1993; 2003; Mittelman *et al.* 1996; Moniz-Cook *et al.* 2009). With increased awareness and improved diagnostics, people with dementia may, in the very early phase of their condition, request or potentially benefit from counselling or psychotherapeutic programmes (Cheston and Howells 2016; Lipinska 2009). Hence, it is necessary to develop and validate psychosocial support programmes that focus specifically on the earlier phases of dementia, when both the person with dementia and their family have to adjust to their diagnosis and changing circumstances (Waldemar *et al.* 2011).

The DAISY study investigated the efficacy of a specialised structured counselling method, designed to meet the needs of recently diagnosed people with mild Alzheimer's disease (AD) and their family. The intervention was developed and applied in the Danish Alzheimer Intervention Study – DAISY, initially carried out at the Danish Dementia Research Centre between 2003 and 2009 and later implemented across several Danish care settings. In the initial single-blind randomised controlled trial, the DAISY intervention was compared with 'usual care' for people with mild, probable AD or mixed AD, who had been diagnosed in the past 12 months and were living at home in close contact with a family carer (see Waldemar *et al.* 2011). Three hundred and thirty people with dementia (151 males and 179 females) and their family carer took part, with 165 allocated to the DAISY intervention group. Average ages of people with dementia and carers were 76 years (range, 54–92 years) and 66 years (range, 22–90 years), respectively. The majority (67%) of family carers were women, 66 per cent were spouses, 26 per cent were adult children or 'in-laws' and 8 per cent had another family relationship. Nearly a third (30.9%) of people with dementia lived alone. The evaluation spanned follow-up at 12 months and three years (Phung *et al.* 2013; Waldorff *et al.* 2012). The main focus of the counselling method is on strengthening positive aspects of life for both the person with dementia and their family carer, and is tailored to each of their potentially differing personal needs and values. DAISY as an intervention has provided healthcare professionals with a new perspective on post-diagnostic counselling and guidance for people with mild dementia and their families.

This chapter outlines in detail the conceptual underpinnings of the counselling intervention and describes the experiences of people with dementia, carers and the counsellors who delivered the programme.

Theoretical aspects: The constructivist socio-dynamic, self-validation counselling model

The approach to counselling allows the person with dementia and the family carer to 'tell his or her life story' and express what is of personal importance to them. Thus it was anchored within participants' positive resources and valued activities, and, for the person with dementia, their retained skills and functions. This approach used the 'constructivist principles' of socio-dynamic counselling (Peavy 1997) and self-validation (Ishiyama 1993), each of which will be considered next in terms of skills required by the counsellor.

Socio-dynamic counselling and 'constructivist' counselling skills in dementia care

Socio-dynamic counselling refers to a general method of life planning to assist individuals to develop their capacities in order to live a valued life, including achieving their pre-defined wishes and goals. It emphasises skills and techniques such as the search for 'meaning' as the person takes responsibility for constructing their own life; the identification and 'validation' of strengths, values and assumptions; and the use of mapping, metaphors and mindfulness in assisting the individual to 'tell their stories'. All counselling models have some value for some people in some contexts and socio-dynamic counselling widens the scope for counselling in dementia care, since it is based on emerging concepts and observations from societies that are in transformation (Peavy 2000).

The counsellor aims to develop a relationship with the person with dementia and the family carer, who are seen experts in their own lives. The relationship is based on the counsellor using language and communication to develop meaningful interaction and engagement with participants. The dialogue for communication necessarily involves listening with inner calmness, harmonious relations, and transformative 'learning'. This allows the counsellor to demonstrate understanding and interest in, or concern for, the person and the family carer. For good dementia care, it is important that the constructivist counsellor takes account of the diagnosis, the danger of trying to achieve 'the unattainable' and the importance of considering both what is valued by the person but is also 'achievable'. Thus in offering support, an individual's life experience, values and strengths are used in conjunction with knowledge of their limitations. The counsellor must be aware of communication as a constructive activity, which will lead to plans and clarity for the person with dementia. Another key dementia-care skill is the counsellor's ability to provide information to the person and the family carer, where the process of understanding may be described as 'transformative learning' – this is an active process, whereby a person with dementia or a family carer makes sense of their new situation by using prior knowledge and making interpretations based on this. The final key skill for good dementia-care counselling is that of a collaborative relationship with the person and the family carer. The constructivist counsellor must make sure there is room for free exchange of information and ideas, with options for innovation. Above all, the counsellor must respect the person with dementia and family carer and take account of the new relationships that are being constructed, following a diagnosis of dementia. Thus counselling must be ethical, meaningful and realistic and thereby:

- create a collaborative working relationship

- view the counselling process as an intelligent 'two-person' team

- use dialogue and combined knowledge or 'intelligence' to develop solutions, new understandings and meaningful action.

Self-validation approaches and techniques: The 'validation-gram'

Self-validation (Ishiyama 1993) is a method for recognising and transcending the sense of self by various means to appreciate the unconditional value and meaning of personal existence. In other words, self-validation is the process of reinforcing or, where needed, restoring the sense of self-worth, meaning of life, personal identity and a sense of competence. This is achieved through a variety of activities and interactions within the person's natural, physical and social environments, where these qualities may also transcend to a creative or spiritual level. Every person is given the lifelong mission of recognising the value of their unique individuality and their collective existence. It is a mission of actualising the potential for attaining the highest form of harmony and peace within oneself, within relationships and within their physical and social environments.

The 'validation-gram' (Ishiyama 1995) allows the counsellor to map views and activities, which are of importance and value to the person or the family carer's life (see Figure 3.1). By putting these matters into words – or illustrations where words are hard to achieve – these can become the subject of conversation, interaction and guidance, when required. Thus the validation-gram is a tool to support a meaningful discussion between the person and the counsellor about the person's own values for a meaningful life. It helps the counsellor to determine how the person's own values can be preserved or restored. The advantages of this approach are that an individual becomes 'visible' and active, and this can facilitate a shared goal between person and counsellor. The method allows people with word-finding or other language difficulties to express themselves through illustrating their values in a variety of ways, including drawings and painting.

The DAISY counselling intervention

Drawing on the constructivist and self-validation principles, the DAISY intervention took account of the particular circumstances of people with dementia and their carers, their wishes for the future and the values that were important to them for a good quality of life. The focus was on strengthening the positive elements of the individual and their networks in everyday life, rather than on problem solving. It was structured to:

- clarify the individual's needs and wishes for support and knowledge

- help align expectations and reach realistic goals, taking into account the capacity of an individual

- promote an understanding of individual and joint situations

- enhance learning on how to seek knowledge and support

- develop individual action plans.

DAISY comprised a series of structured counselling sessions (Table 3.1), including information and support for people with mild dementia as well as their family carers. By offering counselling in the early months following a dementia diagnosis, the aim was to prevent depressive symptoms and further impairments of health-related quality of life in people with dementia and their family carers (see Waldemar *et al.* 2011; Waldorff *et al.* 2012, for a summary of the intervention). The DAISY intervention used four types of counselling sessions, a group-based psycho-educational course where people could also engage with others, and outreach telephone contact.

The intervention began with a structured initial counselling session with both the person and carer and follow-up counselling sessions. A session with the wider family group also occurred, either before or after a two-hour weekly psycho-educational group-based course over five weeks. Two groups were conducted in parallel – one for people with dementia and one for their carers. Thus people with dementia and carers had opportunities for 'peer support'. Individual counselling sessions were planned on an ongoing basis with individuals and their family, while group-based courses were scheduled when sufficient participants had been allocated to the intervention arm of the study. A final counselling session occurred for all people and carers. Regular follow-up outreach telephone contact was used to discuss issues that arose in the individual counselling sessions.

The duration of intervention averaged seven months, ranging from 8 to 12 months (see Søgaard *et al.* 2009). This allowed for tailoring to the needs of the person and the family carer and could be delivered to the person with dementia or the family carer on their own, or together, or carried out as part of a group. The intervention therefore consisted of five key components: counselling sessions; educational courses to provide information about dementia and its consequences and about living and coping with dementia and a forum for people with dementia and families to exchange experiences and coping strategies; written hand-outs; outreach telephone counselling; and log-books (a form of diary) for the person with dementia and/or their family carer. Participants were encouraged to take advantage of all components of the programme.

Table 3.1: DAISY counselling sessions

Session Type	Participants	Agenda	Time schedule
Initial counselling	Counsellor, person with dementia and carer. Counsellor and person with dementia alone. Counsellor and carer alone.	Counsellor follows the structured schedule agenda. Person and carer complete the validation-gram and action plan.	1–1½ hours
Follow-up counselling 2 sessions	Counsellor, person with dementia and carer.	Counsellor follows the structured schedule agenda. Follow-up with both validation-gram and action plan.	20 minutes–1 hour, usually ½ hour
Family counselling	Counsellor, person with dementia, carer and family network.	Counsellor follows the structured schedule agenda. Topics for the meeting gathered from previous conversations.	1–1½ hours
Final counselling	Counsellor, person with dementia alone. Counsellor and carer alone.	Counsellor follows the structured schedule agenda, with follow-up and review of validation-gram and action plan.	1–1½ hours

Counselling sessions

In all counselling sessions the counsellor used a structured interview schedule and a fixed agenda. Each counselling session ended with repetition of the main points of agreement and of any specific needs for supportive activities. Then the counsellor and the dyad agreed on future appointments, such as dates of teaching courses and outreach telephone counselling, which were recorded on a separate form. The counselling sessions were supported by written information and log books kept by the person with dementia and their carer.

Initial counselling

At the first counselling session the person with dementia and carer were given the opportunity to tell their life story and to speak about things that were personally important and of great value to the individual. This was clarified by applying the principles of self-validation and validation-gram (Figure 3.1) as a basis to develop an action plan covering four topics: *Everyday life*, *Relationships with other people*, *Activities*, and *'The best I know'*. The carer completes the validation-gram in a separate room; the person with dementia completes the validation-gram, assisted by the counsellor. The completed validation-gram in DAISY was used in the preparation of an action plan. The counsellor offered participants guidance with decision-making, advice and activities to help participants construct what they perceived as a meaningful life. Written notes were used to focus follow-up sessions with the aim of improving coping strategies and empowering participants to focus on the positive factors and resources in their lives, according to the principles of self-validation.

Follow-up counselling

Face-to-face and outreach phone calls were conducted continuously throughout the intervention period. The interview schedule followed a fixed agenda, ensuring that the objectives of the meeting were achieved. During the session the counsellor talked with the person with dementia and the carer separately and together, with the purpose of adjusting the action plans and validation-grams as required. New needs or problems addressed at follow-up were noted and relevant support activities or contacts were established.

Family counselling

This aimed to clarify the knowledge in the family network about dementia and about the situation of the person affected. Similarly, the purpose of the meeting was to discuss specific concerns and to determine the network resources and the likelihood of getting assistance and support from the family. Family counselling was offered to other family members in addition to the identified primary carer. Family counselling was held after the first counselling session and during the follow-up sessions. Prior to the session, an agenda was discussed together with the person with dementia and the family carer, and it was agreed who would be responsible for bringing up the often differing topics to be discussed during the family counselling session. During the conversation, the counsellor prepared written notes in the form of 'minutes', which summarised agreements and action points. Care was taken not to disclose confidential information about the person with dementia to others in the family without their consent.

Case Study 3.1 – **Mr Hansen**[1]

Mr Hansen is 85 years old and was diagnosed with Alzheimer's disease and prescribed an 'anti-dementia' drug four months ago. He has no physical health complaints other than impaired hearing and has difficulty in accepting that he has dementia. He was an engineer who worked hard throughout his life. His wife is ten years younger than him and in good health. Throughout their marriage, they have always respected each other's interests and differences. The couple have one adult son and one grandchild. They live in a house with a large garden that Mr Hansen has continued to maintain. They used to spend summers at their country cottage but around the time of Mr Hansen's diagnosis of dementia, they sold their cottage in an attempt to simplify responsibilities, such as maintaining upkeep of a second dwelling. However they continue to be upset at the loss of their longstanding pleasurable summer routines at their cottage. Mrs Hansen has difficulty in acknowledging the consequences of her husband's dementia and in adjusting to manage their new life circumstances.

After the first counselling session, the couple began to accept the new situation and developed an action plan (see Figure 3.1 for

---

1   A pseudonym.

Mr Hansen's value-based validation-gram; and Table 3.2 for his action plan). Their next counselling session was scheduled for two months' time.

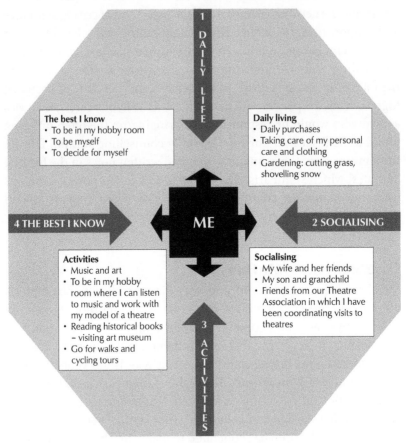

Figure 3.1: Mr Hansen's validation-gram

Table 3.2: Mr Hansen's action plan

Topic	Conclusion	Distribution of tasks (CR – counsellor)
Knowledge about: • dementia • medication • legal advice	Was offered to join a training course targeted to people living with dementia. Refuses because he could not see the need for this.	CR ensures knowledge of dementia is given in an acceptable way during individual sessions ensuring that Mr Hansen understands his changing circumstances due to declining cognition.

Topic	Conclusion	Distribution of tasks (CR – counsellor)
Daily living • Practical tasks • Personal care • Safety • Medical care • Shopping	There is no need for help with personal care and practical tasks in the house and garden. Mr Hansen often forgets to take his 'anti-dementia' medication since he has always been healthy.	His wife agrees to support her husband in remembering to take his medicine.
Routines and habits • Day • Night	No need for support.	
Getting around • Uses his bike and public transport • Orientation • Physical ability good – he can walk, run, etc.	Mr Hansen values going for walks and cycling; but he often gets lost, which has reduced these pleasurable activities.	To maintain the walking and cycling, CR requests the Municipality for a GPS that gives Mr Hansen increased security and freedom of movement and helps his wife to locate him if necessary. CR guides Mr Hansen and his wife on how to use the GPS.
• **When**	When Mr Hansen is in his hobby room he has a sense of harmony and joy.	Mrs Hansen encourages him to maintain activities in the hobby room. His son and grandchild all encourage this by joining him in the hobby room when they visit.
Nutrition • Cooking • Appetite • Diet • Weight	No need for support.	
The future • Economic conditions • Legal planning • Who helps	The couple to consider together power of attorney to allow Mr Hansen to name his wife to make financial and other decisions in the future if needed.	The couple have always had independent bank accounts. Now Mrs Hansen is engaged in managing their finances and helps her husband with his banking tasks, when he feels he needs this.
Activities and hobbies	The couple have never travelled. Mr Hansen would like to travel with his wife.	The couple have started travelling abroad.

cont.

Topic	Conclusion	Distribution of tasks (CR – counsellor)
Need for help • Nurse • Homecare • Activity centre • Getting around • Assistive products	No need for support.	
Network contacts • Closest relatives • Family • Friends • Neighbours • Other	Socialising is important for Mr Hansen, particularly his relationships with his son, grandchild and friends. He feels that his friends from the theatre group are withdrawing from their friendship with him.	CR invites the son to join the next meeting where they discuss tips and ideas to how to extend and reinforce contact, including with the grandchild so they can have fun and joy together. CR guides the couple on ways of sharing the diagnosis and its current effects with friends and also ways of engaging their support and maintaining their relationships.

Qualifications and training of counsellors

The counsellor needs knowledge and skills in communication and education to act as a future 'lifeline' for the person with dementia, the identified carer and the wider family network. To provide good counselling requires loyalty, flexibility and creativity and demonstration of commitment, knowledge and interest. Timing, empathy and intuition are also important. The characteristics of a skilled counsellor include maturity and responsibility, but also the ability to recognise one's own limitations; for example, by involving other professionals when necessary. As a counsellor one may be inclined to sway the advice in a particular direction and perhaps choose the advice that one believes would be best for other people. In this context, the counsellor must be aware of whether they are applying indirect authority.

The DAISY counsellors were all specialist nurses with several years of experience in dementia care and in counselling. Prior to the study they participated in a four-day course to learn about the basic concepts of interventions with people with dementia and carers, and the objectives of this particular method of counselling. Training also contained formal teaching about communication and counselling drawing on constructivist principles and methodology. Throughout the intervention period, the study coordinators were offered supervision on a regular basis within eight centralised follow-up sessions and regular site visits from the team coordinating the study.

Outcomes

Semi-structured interviews with a sub-sample of 11 couples selected from the 165 dyads randomised to the DAISY intervention were conducted before and one to three months after the intervention (Sørensen *et al.* 2008). These were conducted separately with the carer and the person with dementia. In the first interview, participants were asked to describe their experiences in the following domains: daily activities; recent changes in daily activities; and social relations with spouse/relative, family and friends. In the second interview, participants were asked to describe the same domains and to highlight any recent changes; in addition, they were asked to describe their personal experiences of the intervention.

The tailored counselling appeared to provide opportunities for carers to engage in early reflections that altered attitudes and coping efficacy through an understanding of dementia. During and after the intervention, they reported improved coping with the challenges of the dementia and felt better able to face everyday life and social relations with more serenity and competence. They also appreciated receiving important information, support on how to cope with the consequences of the disease, and guidance on maintaining wellbeing. The intervention appeared to provide opportunities for people with dementia and families to appreciate different aspects of their own situations and to receive support from peers and professionals (Sørensen *et al.* 2008).

Focus groups were conducted to gather data on the experiences of the counsellors. A selection of comments from these and from the interviews with study participants are shown in the box below.

Comments from Spouse 1:

'I have become confident about the situation. I know what to do when the different situations occur, I know who to contact, and that is a great help. If there is something I don't know I can look it up in my book. The intervention has given me the information I need; it is a great help that I don't have to search for it myself. I have also learned how to take care of myself and how to preserve my energy. I have become more pragmatic. I don't feel guilty when I need a break, so I take it when I am getting exhausted, when I get palpitations or stomach ache.'

Comment from Person with dementia A:

'This is the first time I feel someone is listening to me.'

Comment from Person with dementia B:

'It was very nice in the groups. Not everybody liked going there at first, but later everybody was enthusiastic. If somebody said something stupid we took it as a joke. It is a pity it stopped; we could continue to talk and support each other. I would like to continue in that group because there I don´t feel stupid when I can´t remember the words – it is easier to talk to others who have similar difficulties as I have.'

Comment from Spouse 2:

'During the counselling I learned that I get valuable support from regular contact with a professional counsellor, and I appreciate having established a contact for the future. I have also joined a permanent support group for carers and there I talk about subjects I can't discuss with...[spouse]'

Counsellor comments on the intervention:

'The individual consultations provided a greater openness in the family and the person with dementia felt heard.'
'I must be professionally prepared but also be in possession of personal qualities and impact.'

'It can be difficult to "separate" the person with dementia and the carer during the counselling sessions which were separate for them – I needed a task to give to them.'

'To start using the validation-gram was a great challenge.'

'I had to remind myself about getting eye contact with the person with dementia.'

The counselling sessions were evaluated using a questionnaire, which was completed by 63 per cent of people with dementia and carers (Table 3.3). The majority were very satisfied with the approach to counselling that was used.

Table 3.3: Evaluation of DAISY counselling by people with dementia and carers

Counselling where you've been alone with the counsellor: What was your overall impression of the counselling sessions?[1]						
	Very good	Good	Less good	Not good	Don't know	Not participated
PwD* (N = 103)	42%	44%	3%	1%	8%	2%
Carer (N = 104)	58%	36%	2%	-	1%	3%

Counselling where you've been together with the counsellor. What was your overall impression of the counselling sessions?[2]						
	Very good	Good	Less good	Not good	Don't know	Not participated
PwD (N = 103)	41%	50%	1%	1%	7%	
Carer (N = 104)	47%	48%	1%	-	3%	1%

Counselling where you've all been together with your family and the counsellor. What was your overall impression of the counselling sessions?[3]						
	Very good	Good	Less good	Not good	Don't know	Not participated
PwD (N = 103)	27%	32%	6%	-	4%	31%
Carer (N = 104)	34%	32%	3%	-	2%	29%

*PwD – Person with dementia [1]with counsellor alone; [2]with counsellor and designated primary (family) carer; [3]with counsellor, designated family carer and wider family network

The randomised controlled trial demonstrated some gains managing depression and in family perception of quality of life of their relative, when compared to the 'control condition' (Waldorff *et al.* 2012), although these were not maintained at three-year follow-up (Phung *et al.* 2013). Of note is that control intervention was far in excess of 'usual care' in Denmark, comprising three visits by an interviewer who referred the person and/or the carer to local support activities when needed. There were no significant negative outcomes or adverse events related to the intervention.

There were some caveats to our somewhat intensive approach to intervention. First, people and families were invited to join regardless of their expected or expressed need for this particular support. Thus the intervention was not restricted to people actively seeking assistance. Second, participation in the DAISY intervention group was seen as quite demanding for some carers as well as for some people with dementia. Third, adherence to the many counselling meetings and courses was difficult for some, particularly those with health problems, or for busy carers, and for those living some distance away from the study centre. We noted that although not participating in the intensive intervention we designed, the control group was also seen by researchers, where some families spoke about their emerging psychosocial and health problems and were supported to access available resources and relevant health professionals. Thus, based on the experiences and outcomes in the DAISY study, we recommend that people with dementia and carers with more symptoms and 'greater need' should be offered the full intensive intervention programme, and that regular follow-up to determine support needs may be sufficient for those who have minimal symptoms and needs at the time of diagnosis.

Implementation and conclusions

Several Danish municipalities have implemented the counselling model and the courses in their services for people with dementia and their carers. The first implementation project in a municipality near Copenhagen received a very positive evaluation from both quantitative and qualitative data. People with dementia as well as their carers were very happy with the support and education provided. The dementia coordinators who carried out the counselling sessions and the courses also had viewed this more structured way of working as a better way of providing support than other less structured methods of support that some might use to support people with dementia and carers. During 2014, this counselling model remained the preferred method for supporting people with dementia and their carers in the Municipality of Lyngby-Taarbæk close to Copenhagen. Five dementia coordinators were educated using the counselling model and they continue to provide the intervention at the time of writing (2019).

In early 2017, The National Dementia Action Plan, *A Safe and Dignified Life with Dementia,* was published in Denmark.[2] The action plan sets out three national targets for dementia efforts until 2025. This is supported by 23 clear initiatives, where Initiative 11 covers the 'Development and dissemination of a national toolbox with patient and relative courses'. This focuses on support and counselling for relatives of people with dementia by development of a national toolbox including information material and well-tried tools for establishing and implementing courses and group opportunities for people with dementia and carers. The DAISY counselling programme that has been described in this chapter is, amongst others, an example of counselling approaches that are included in the Initiative 11 toolbox.

References

Brodaty, H., Green, A. and Koschera, A. (2003) 'Meta-analysis of psychosocial interventions for caregivers of people with dementia.' *Journal of the American Geriatric Society 51*, 657–664.

Brodaty, H., McGilchrist, C., Harris, L. and Peters, K.E. (1993) 'Time until institutionalization and death in patients with dementia: Role of caregiver training and risk factors.' *Archives of Neurology 50*, 643–650.

Cheston, R. and Howells, L. (2016) 'A feasibility study of translating "Living Well with Dementia" groups into a primary care improving access to psychological therapy service (innovative practice).' *Dementia 15*, 2, 273–278.

Ishiyama, F.I. (1993) 'On self-validation.' *The Trumpeter, Journal of Ecosophy 10*, 2–8.

Ishiyama, F.I. (1995) 'Use of validation-gram in counseling: Exploring sources of self-validation and impact of personal transition.' *Canadian Journal of Counseling/Revue canadienne de counselling 29*, 2, 134–146.

Lipinska, D. (2009) *Person-Centred Counselling for People with Dementia: Making Sense of Self.* London: Jessica Kingsley Publishers.

Mittelman, M.S., Ferris, S.H., Shulman, E., Steinberg, G. and Levin, B. (1996) 'A family intervention to delay nursing home placement of patients with Alzheimer disease: A randomized controlled trial.' *Journal of American Medical Association 276*, 1725–1731.

Moniz-Cook, E., Gibson, G., Harrison, J. and Wilkinson, H. (2009) 'Timely Psychosocial Interventions in a Memory Clinic.' In E. Moniz-Cook and J. Manthorpe (eds) *Early*

2   www.sum.dk/Temaer/National%20demenshandlingsplan.aspx

Psychosocial Interventions in Dementia: Evidence-based Practice. London: Jessica Kingsley Publishers.

Peavy, V.R. (1997) *SocioDynamic Counselling: A Constructivist Perspective for the Practice of Counselling in the 21st Century.* Victoria, BC: Trafford Publishing.

Peavy, V. (2000) *PART 1: A Brief Outline of SocioDynamic Counselling: A Co-Constructivist Perspective on Helping,* Revised 24 May 2001. Accessed on 16/10/2019 at www.sociodynamic-constructivist-counselling.com/documents/brief_outline.pdf

Phung, K.T.T., Waldorff, F.B., Buss, D.V., Eckermann, A. *et al.* (2013) 'A three-year follow-up on the efficacy of psychosocial interventions for patients with mild dementia and their caregivers: The multicentre, rater-blinded, randomised Danish Alzheimer Intervention Study (DAISY).' *British Medical Journal Open 3,* e003584.

Søgaard. R., Sørensen, J., Waldorff, F.B., Eckermann, A. *et al.* (2009) 'Private costs almost equal health care costs when intervening in mild Alzheimer's: A cohort study alongside the DAISY trial.' *BMC Health Services Research 9,* 215.

Sørensen, LV., Waldorff, F.B. and Waldemar, G. (2008) 'Early counselling and support for patients with mild Alzheimer's disease and their caregivers: A qualitative study on outcome.' *Aging & Mental Health 12,* 444–450.

Waldemar, G., Waldorff, F.B., Buss, D.V., Eckermann, A. *et al.* (2011) 'The Danish Alzheimer Intervention Study: Rationale, study design and baseline characteristics of the cohort.' *Neuroepidemiology 36,* 52–61.

Waldorff, F.B., Buss, D.V., Eckermann, A., Rasmussen, M.L. *et al.* (2012) 'Efficacy of psychosocial intervention in patients with mild Alzheimer's disease: The multicentre, rater blinded, randomised Danish Alzheimer Intervention Study (DAISY).' *British Medical Journal 345,* e4693. doi:10.1136/bmj.e4693

Related reading

Antonovsky, A. (1987) *Unravelling the Mystery of Health: How People Manage Stress and Stay Well.* San Francisco, CA: Jossey-Bass.

Søgaard, R., Sørensen, J., Waldorff, F., B., Eckermann, A. *et al.* (2014) 'Early psychosocial intervention in Alzheimer's disease: Cost utility evaluation alongside the Danish Alzheimer's Intervention Study (DAISY).' *British Medical Journal Open 4,* 1, e004105. doi:10.1136/bmjopen-2013-004105.

Sørensen, L.V., Waldorff, F.B. and Waldemar, G. (2008) 'Coping with mild Alzheimer's disease.' *Dementia 7,* 287–299.

Sørensen, L.V., Waldorff, F.B. and Waldemar, G. (2007) 'Social participation in home-living patients with mild Alzheimer's disease.' *Archives of Gerontology and Geriatrics 47,* 291–301.

Waldorff, F.B., Nielsen, A.B.S. and Waldemar, G. (2010) 'Self-rated health in patients with mild Alzheimer's disease: Baseline data from the Danish Alzheimer Intervention Study.' *Archives of Gerontology and Geriatrics 50,* 1–5.

Chapter 4

Meeting Centres and Dementia Cafés

COMMUNITY-BASED INITIATIVES AND SOCIAL ENGAGEMENT

Rose-Marie Dröes, Rabih Chattat and Stefanie Auer

Introduction

Dementia has a major impact on the lives of people and their families, but people often postpone asking for help due to reasons such as the persisting taboo and stigma of dementia, poor expectations of post-diagnostic services, and fears of dependency or having to move to a care home. Fragmentation of care services further hampers the scope for people and families to find support.

In the last two decades community-based services and social support programmes have begun to address these constraints across Europe. Such programmes include the Meeting Centres Support Programme (MCSP), Alzheimer Cafés, the Dementia Service Centres (DSC) initiative and the Bistrot Mémoire. There are several commonalities across these innovations. First is that they offer support in an easily accessible, socially integrated context, with a focus on both people with dementia and their family or other carers. Second is the active involvement of the person with dementia throughout the communication and information processes and in contributing to the choice of the range of activities that are organised. This aspect of social inclusion reflects respect for, and recognition of, people with dementia within these facilities. Third is their scope to work together closely with other care and welfare agencies and organisations and professionals that deliver support to people with dementia living at home and their carers. These factors, alongside ongoing publicity to increase public awareness about the importance of timely support in dementia, are mechanisms whereby uptake of relevant services, social inclusion and wellbeing for the person living with dementia can be enhanced. They can also reduce carer stress and contribute to the de-stigmatisation of dementia. The intensive collaboration with other services that is implicit in such initiatives has the added advantage of counteracting fragmentation of care and support services. Dissemination has been promoted by manuals on how to set up such a service, staff training, informative websites, service-related research and ongoing publicity. Carers and people with dementia themselves promote dissemination as seen by their high levels of take-up and appreciation of these initiatives.

The Meeting Centres Support Programme (MCSP) and Alzheimer Café approach both originated in The Netherlands. They are perhaps most widely disseminated across Europe. The MCSP has been described in detail (Dröes, Meiland and van Tilburg 2006a; Dröes *et al.* 2011) and has been rigorously evaluated for effectiveness (Dröes *et al.* 2000; 2004a; 2006b) and implementation into practice in The Netherlands (Dröes *et al.* 2004b; Meiland *et al.* 2005; Smits *et al.* 2007). Recently a pan-European collaboration, the MEETINGDEM project (2014–2017)[1] has systematically examined the implementation of this programme in centres in Italy, Poland and the UK (Dröes *et al.* 2017).

This chapter will first summarise the MCSP template, and will discuss its adaptive implementation in the MEETINGDEM study. This will be followed by a description of Meeting Places in one region of Italy, where the Meeting Centres model was implemented in a less intensive manner and combined with an Alzheimer Café approach. Next we will describe two similar initiatives that have emerged as accessible, post-diagnostic support programmes across Europe (i.e. the Bistrot Mémoire in France, Dementia Service Centres in Austria), and in the US (i.e. Memory Clubs and Brookdale Respite Programme, which are probably the two most widely disseminated support programmes for people with dementia and carers in the US). The chapter will conclude by summarising some key elements of these programmes, their potential for implementation in different contexts and cultures, and recommendations for research.

---

1   www.meetingdem.eu

Meeting Centres Support Programme
The approach

Meeting Centres, originally established in Amsterdam in 1993, offer support for home-dwelling people with mild to moderate dementia and their carers. People with dementia participate in a *social club* (held three days each week), where a small professional team (two professionals for 12–15 participants) and volunteers (one per day) offer a range of *activities*, such as playing games, singing, shopping, preparing lunch, cognitive stimulation, reminiscence, arts-based activities and psychomotor therapy. The carer can attend *discussion groups* and a series of *information sessions*, covering subjects such as dementia, dealing with behaviour changes and available support services. The meeting centre offers *case management*, a weekly *consultation hour* and *social activities* for both people with dementia and carers. Regular meetings are organised, where all participants (people with dementia and carers), staff and volunteers, discuss the activities, in order to better attune them to the needs and wishes of the participants. In this way the joint commitment to their Meeting Centre (often described as 'the Club' by participants) is strengthened.

A psychosocial 'care diagnosis' (or needs assessment), consisting of information on unmet needs, adaptation and coping problems and participants' wishes, provides the basis for an 'individualised needs-directed' support strategy. Based on the support strategy and the person's preferences for types of activities, an individually tailored activity plan is drawn up for each person with dementia. Support strategies for carers vary according to their needs and wishes, ranging from providing information, to practical, emotional and/or social support.

The outcomes

Studies show that, compared to nursing-home-based day care without carer support, the MCSP is more successful in delaying institutionalisation and reducing levels of inactivity, behavioural problems and depression in people with dementia, while improvements in self-esteem are also noted (Dröes *et al.* 2000; 2004a, 2004b). Carers report feeling more competent and less burdened (Dröes *et al.* 2004a), and those who are lonely report fewer psychosomatic complaints than carers using day care only as a form of respite (Meiland *et al.* 2010). Overall, participants are highly satisfied with the Meeting Centres

(Dröes *et al.* 2011). One reason for this may be that they are integrated into local community facilities that allow shared social activities (e.g. playing billiards or having a drink at the bar) with other visitors. This can enhance local connections, help recruit volunteers and counteract the stigma of dementia.

When cognitive impairments become severe, making it difficult for people to participate in group activities within a community centre, another setting for the person must be arranged, for example at home, day care or a long-term care facility. Some Meeting Centres avoid such moves by organising different rooms with activities and social support to match the 'stage' of decline in a person with dementia.

Implementation

To stimulate dissemination and offer ideas about what helps in the successful implementation of Meeting Centres a practical manual was prepared (Dröes and Van Ganzewinkel 2015). Meeting Centres are usually set up by a group of local stakeholders such as home care providers, GPs, the local memory clinic or mental health service, local welfare or social care service and the Alzheimer Association, one of which takes on the responsibility of recruiting staff. Over a six- to nine-month period, small working groups make all necessary preparations for the new Meeting Centre. They take account of the aims of the meeting service, staff training, location and funding, and develop a collaborative protocol with other services. This programme is now widely available across The Netherlands, where, since 2017, some 145 Meeting Centres are in operation.

MEETINGDEM aimed to evaluate translation of the MCSP to three European countries, namely Italy, Poland and the UK (Dröes *et al.* 2017). After exploring pathways to care in each country, translation involved: establishing a group of organisational collaborators and user representatives; outlining facilitators and barriers to implementing MCSP in each setting; establishing implementation plans; developing practical guides and toolkits by adapting the Dutch materials to local requirements; and training staff. Nine Meeting Centres were initially established in Italy (5), Poland (2) and the UK (2); and later another further four in Italy and two in Poland. The first nine participated in a study (see Dröes *et al.* 2017) designed to examine MCSPs' impact on people with dementia and carers and also their cost-effectiveness. In summarising the results it can be concluded that MCSP is transferable across countries, showing improvements in aspects of quality of life and mental health benefits for people with dementia and carers against small additional costs.

MEETINGDEM evaluation

Overall the MCSP concept and components were maintained in all countries and centres. Country-specific requirements resulted in variations in inclusion criteria, frequency of programme components and culture-specific activities. Factors facilitating implementation were: added value of MCSP and evidence of its effectiveness; matching needs of the target group; enthusiastic local stakeholders; suitable staff and project manager. Barriers were: competition with other care/welfare organisations and limited funding.

The evaluation comparing MCSP with usual care in the three countries showed that MCSP was more effective for promoting feelings of belonging, self-esteem and positive affect in people with dementia (with medium to large effect sizes). Higher attendance was associated with increased feelings of support reported by people with dementia, and higher reduction in reported neuropsychiatric symptoms. Carers experienced less stress than those receiving usual care. In Italy, carers' mood improved and they were less distressed.

The economic evaluation showed that compared to 'standard day care centres' the combined MCSP costs only 3 euro/hour more (20%). Emerging findings suggest that for some quality of life in dementia measures (i.e. QOL-AD, DQoL), MCSP may be cost-effective.

People with dementia and carers were highly satisfied with MCSP. Carers reported that the activities for people with dementia were functionally 'activating' and provide an important means for social and emotional interaction.

Adaptive implementation of MCSP in other European countries has also occurred (Brooker, Dröes and Evans 2017; Brooker *et al.* 2018; Mangiaracina *et al.* 2017; Szcześniak *et al.* 2018 and Westerman *et al.* 2017).

In the next section we describe a precursor to MEETINGDEM in one region of Italy (Emilia-Romagna), where, to contextualise support to local stakeholders the Meeting Centres and Alzheimer Café (Miesen and Jones 2004) were combined.

Meeting Places in Italy
Background and approach

Meeting Places in Italy are a combination of Alzheimer Cafés and the Meeting Centre approach. Alzheimer Cafés, using the format suggested by the Dutch psychologist Bere Miesen (Miesen and Jones 2004), were introduced in Italy in 2003. The first Alzheimer Cafés were used mostly by family carers although a few people with dementia also attended. Lack of participation by people with dementia was thought to be due to country differences associated with disclosure of the diagnosis and involvement of the person with dementia in discussion of their disease. This was more common in The Netherlands compared to Italy where at that time diagnostic disclosure involving the person with dementia was relatively rare.

In 2005, the Emilia-Romagna regional dementia plan recognised the Alzheimer Café as an intervention that should be available for people with dementia and their carers, but there were no guidelines on how this should happen. In 2007, a first Meeting Centre-type initiative was launched combining the existing Alzheimer Café approach with the Meeting Centres model. The aim of this Meeting Place was to reduce social isolation across the stages of dementia, by offering discussions and meaningful activities such as mental stimulation and recreational activities, out of the home, for people with dementia and carers. In 2009 a description of the basic structure and content of the initiative was published on the regional website.[2] The main characteristics of Meeting Places in this part of Italy are:

- open access for any person with dementia and carer

- involvement of volunteers in the activities

- once a week three-hour sessions with meaningful activities for people with dementia and carers

- support from other local agencies with matters such as transport or other resources

- the presence of two people with training in dementia support, with responsibility for the activities

---

2   http://sociale.regione.emilia-romagna.it/documentazione/pubblicazioni/guide/
dicafeincafeguida.pdf/view

- the availability, on request, of other experts to talk to members of the group or to discuss matters that arise.

The outcomes

In 2011 a pre-post pilot study over six months was conducted of the Meeting Places in Italy. This involved 31 people with dementia and 35 carers. A reduction in behavioural symptoms in people with dementia and reduced levels of social and emotional burden in carers were found. There were also indications from interviews with people with dementia and carers that Meeting Places are helpful in building new relationships and reducing social isolation.

Spouse: 'At the meeting place she [wife] takes part in the activities, while at home she is not active.'

Person with dementia: 'I feel better at the meeting place, I had a nice afternoon with beautiful people. For me it is a familiar place, we can talk, we do things together, we are with other people. I enjoy a lot spending time with other people.'

Person with dementia: 'The meeting place is a place where we are kindly accepted, at the beginning it was not easy, then it becomes helpful and now I don't feel myself alone.'

Carer: 'We become friends with other families... We have the same problems so we feel close to each other. We meet also outside the meeting place.'

Implementation

Meeting Places have become an acceptable approach to improve the social inclusion of people with dementia and their carers in Italy. In 2016 there were 84 Meeting Places in the region of Emilia-Romagna, mostly organised by Alzheimer Associations collaborating with health and social services. The model has also spread to other Italian regions, with a similar basic structure and a high degree of flexibility, in order to meet local needs.

Meeting Places offer participants learning opportunities across the course of dementia through contacts with others, including experts. Furthermore, the Meeting Place can be seen as a 'bottom-up' process, drawing on resources at different levels ranging from the voluntary sector to health and social care agencies. This also empowers families to play an active part in a local Meeting Place.

Alzheimer Cafés
The approach

The concept of an Alzheimer Café was originally developed in The Netherlands in 1997 by Miesen (Miesen and Jones 2004). The aims of the Alzheimer Café are to provide a space and the opportunity for people with dementia and their relatives to speak openly about dementia and other related problems and to receive information about dementia; and to prevent social isolation of people living with dementia and their families.

An Alzheimer Café takes place every month. It usually begins with participants having coffee or tea, followed by a presentation or talk by an expert. After an interval with music and drinks, people with dementia and carers can exchange experiences and ask for information about different aspects of care. The meeting ends informally with general conversation and refreshments. Each meeting generally lasts around two and a half hours. To emphasise that they are part of a local community, the Cafés are organised in community-based settings and people can attend when they wish.

The outcomes

Cafés were a new kind of support for persons with dementia and their carers. Despite the success of the format and its take-up elsewhere, little research has been conducted to assess the outcomes. The literature mainly consists of describing different settings and initiatives (see for example Mather 2006). Capus (2005) suggests that the café experience has an impact on social isolation, provides the opportunity to exchange experiences and information on available services, and is perceived to be a safe space where the experience of dementia can be reformulated. An Australian study (Dow *et al.* 2011) found that an Alzheimer Café promotes social inclusion and emotional wellbeing.

Implementation

The format of an Alzheimer Café has been widely disseminated, first in The Netherlands and later adapted to local contexts and resources in the UK, Ireland, Australia and Canada. Different names are used, for example Kingston Dementia Café (Capus 2005), Poppy Café (Halley *et al.* 2005) in the UK, and the Memory Lane Café in Australia (Dow *et al.* 2011) Initially, Alzheimer Cafés were set up as particularly suitable for people in the early stage of dementia. In practice, however, each country and context has developed their own access protocols. Similarly, the type of programme offered and the role of the other participants can differ between countries. Some involve volunteers or other social organisations. However, all Café initiatives appear to share the overall plan and goals to use a community-based setting, with open access and an informal atmosphere, where people with dementia and carers can discuss and share experiences and information.

An Alzheimer Café helps to promote social inclusion and 'normalise' experiences for both people with dementia and carers. Accessibility of a Café is an important aspect since the initiative can be tailored to people with dementia in different stages of the disease. This implies that different programmes must be offered, moving from information and discussion towards various activities and tailoring the time of the meeting and its duration to meet the needs of the target group.

The popularity of the idea of running Cafés is remarkably high, which is not surprising as they are easily adaptable to different contexts and are relatively inexpensive ways of harnessing resources from different agencies.

Bistrot Mémoire in France
The approach

The first *Bistrot Mémoire* (memory café) in France was launched in Rennes in 2004. In 2012 one hundred participants took part in the national meeting of Bistrots Mémoire in Nantes (see Penna 2012). In 2017 around 50 Bistrots Mémoire appear on the national website.[3] Coulon and Sipos (2013) note that the Bistrot Mémoire is not a place that provides information about the different aspects of the disease is, but a place where people with dementia and their family carers

---

3   www.bistrot-memoire.com

can exchange and share their experiences, opinions and ideas about dementia and related aspects, with others in similar circumstances and with professionals.

The Bistrots take place in a public context, generally a normal bistrot or restaurant, usually during the afternoon once a week (or twice a month), depending on resources and geographical area, for three hours. To ensure the quality of the meeting the activities in the Bistrot are supported by an expert (usually a psychologist) and trained volunteers. Participants are free to join in a part or the whole session.

During the session, a brief lecture or talk is given about a specific topic to promote debate and discussion between all participants. This can be given by an expert, a participant or a guest speaker. The topics are not necessarily dementia-related, other subjects are also discussed. Recreational or leisure activities can also be part of the programme, including external activities, such as trips out.

The outcomes

No research has yet been undertaken on the outcomes of the Bistrots Mémoire, but Coulon and Sipos (2013) have described their background, mission and objectives, basic activities, preconditions and the type and role of participants, especially the experts and volunteers. This detailed description can be seen as a modelling phase of the intervention.

The rapid diffusion of the Bistrots Mémoire in France, and of Alzheimer Cafés in other countries (such as The Netherlands, UK, Italy and Australia), means that evaluation is needed to gain better understanding of their potential for socialisation and participation of people with dementia and their potential role in reducing the stigma of dementia. Their policy of having open access for people with dementia without any previous assessment, their provision of 'normal' or ordinary activities, their role in providing opportunities to discuss and share ideas with others, can all be seen as ways to stimulate inclusion and recognition.

Implementation

The Bistrots Mémoire were initially set up in the west of France, and a national alliance was established with a website offering information about the concept, how to set up or find a Bistrot and opportunity to share initiatives and events.

Dementia Service Centres in Austria
The approach

A Dementia Service Centre (DSC) is a multicomponent, low-threshold, 'one-stop shop' psychosocial support model, specifically addressing the needs of people with dementia and their family carers and support providers (Auer, Span and Reisberg 2015). In this long-term support model the main goals are:

- early disease detection

- diagnostic counselling (support during the process of receiving a diagnosis)

- the development of a positive life-concept as well as the prevention of premature institutionalisation

- carer support.

All elements of the treatment model are developed in a stage-specific fashion (Reisberg *et al.* 1982) in order to provide the right service at the right time. The main treatment elements are the stage-specific training for the person with dementia, and the training and support for care providers. For the care provider, five training modules have been developed. Since mid-2017, eight DSCs are active in Austria, with data available for seven of these. People who approach a DSC for support receive a baseline evaluation and, if eligible, are registered on a longitudinal database, which dates back to 2001, and they are monitored annually with a standard assessment protocol.

The outcomes

A three-and-a-half-year exploratory controlled study was conducted of the DSCs. A total of 141 dyads of people with dementia and support providers were contacted about taking part in the study. People with dementia (N = 83) who met the inclusion criteria were randomised to either the treatment or the control 'treatment as usual' group. The study showed a trend towards disease stabilisation for the treatment group on the Global Deterioration Scale, the Mini Mental State Examination and the Functional Assessment Staging Test (Auer *et al.* 2015). Other studies have focused on acceptance of the service and on subjective carer 'burden' (Mechtler 2008), where two thirds (66%; N = 144) reported a reduction of subjective burden. The majority of carers (85%; N = 157) were satisfied with the DSC service. On average, families used the service for nearly two (1.9) years, with one family involved for over 14 years.

In September 2016, the database contained data of 3681 people with dementia (mean age = 77.69 years) of whom two thirds were female (N = 2461; 66%). About 60 per cent (N = 2298) of registered individuals entered the services of the DSCs without a dementia diagnosis and were, if the psychological test results were indicative of possible dementia, referred to a medical specialist. More than half (53%) of those registered on the database (N = 1959) had participated in at least one stage-specific training programme; 907 (24%) had subsequently died and 785 (21%) had moved to a care home.

Implementation

The DSCs are currently located in rural, difficult-to-serve areas, but more recently also in urban areas. They are located in easily accessible, environmentally appealing venues within a community. A DSC is run by a team consisting of a social worker (30 hours a week) and a psychologist (20 hours a week). Both professionals coordinate and supervise a group of about ten trainers per DSC. These trainers work either in the DSC or in the region where the person lives (see Schulz *et al.* 2012). Extensive public relations efforts are undertaken to increase awareness of dementia. The DSCs hold events that are open to the general public in order to promote social solidarity and facilitate social inclusion of persons with dementia. There is close collaboration with other care professionals and care organisations in order to prevent service fragmentation. To clarify all support processes within the DSC model, a manual is provided to all staff and organisations setting up further DSCs. The DSC model is currently (mid-2017) ready to roll out with funding from the state insurance of Upper Austria and is a centrepiece of the Austrian Dementia Strategy.

Memory Clubs in the US

The approach

A Memory Club targets people with early-stage dementia and their carers with the aim to enhance discussion and participation between the person with dementia and their family carer in an emotionally supportive atmosphere. The approach is based on traditional family therapy where the objective is to strengthen the relationship between couples or between parents and adult children. The main objectives of a Club are to:

- provide information about the disease and resources for coping with it

- improve communication skills

- strengthen the relationship between family members

- reduce the stigma through increased efforts to reach out to other family members and friends

- improve the ability to plan future decisions.

A Memory Club programme consists of 10 to 13 weekly sessions lasting 90 to 120 minutes. Each session is moderated by two facilitators. Half of each session is devoted to topics that involve the entire group, and half is spent in separate peer groups: one for people with memory loss and one for their partners or carers. The session ends with a joint closing activity.

The programme aims to reduce social isolation among people with dementia and carers, enhance self efficacy and the ability to address care issues, and promote communication between members of the dyad and with others. Other expected outcomes are improved wellbeing, awareness of difficulties in the care for the person with dementia, and knowledge about support services and interventions.

The outcomes

Several feasibility and implementation studies of Memory Clubs have been conducted in the last decade, although all lacked a control comparison group (Gaugler *et al.* 2011; Logsdon *et al.* 2010; Zarit *et al.* 2004). The main outcomes demonstrated through these evaluations for the people with dementia are improved Instrumental Activities of Daily Living, as reported by carers; and for the carers enhanced perceived effectiveness in caring. Carers' satisfaction with the Memory Club was high and they reported that they would recommend it to other carers. People with dementia were moderately satisfied and they would also recommend the activities to others with dementia. Discussing their study results, Gaugler and colleagues (2011) underlined the most important benefits of participation in the Memory Club as being:

- availability of information and education of partners in preparing for the future

- improvement of their competence in dealing with care tasks

- confidence in managing memory loss.

Several factors influenced the results, such as the person with dementia's level of cognitive impairment and differences between the study sites.

Implementation

Memory Clubs are currently being held at different locations throughout the US, such as in Minnesota/Dakota (see Alzheimer's Association[4]).

The Brookdale National Group Respite Program in the US

The approach

Since 1989, the Brookdale Foundation's National Group Respite Program has supported community-based organisations in developing and implementing social group activities and respite programmes. These day programmes have spread across the US and have served large numbers of older people with Alzheimer's disease or related dementia and their family carers and also include programmes for people with Early Memory Loss.

The goals of the activities and respite programmes (as summarised by the Brookdale Foundation website[5]) are:

- to offer opportunities for persons with Alzheimer's disease or a related dementia to engage in a program of meaningful social and recreational activities in a secure and supportive setting in order to maximize their cognitive and social abilities

---

4   www.alz.org/mnnd/in_my_community_56782.asp
5   www.brookdalefoundation.net/Respite/respiteprogram.html

- to provide relief and support to family members and other primary caregivers of individuals with Alzheimer's disease or a related dementia.

In addition to providing enjoyable group activities, that build on the strengths and abilities of people with dementia, and respite care, the programmes also offer various other types of support for family carers, such as counselling, support groups, information and referral to other health and social services, training and education. The main objective of the programmes for Early Memory Loss is to offer people with Mild Cognitive Impairment and early-stage dementia the opportunity to learn practical skills in a non-threatening group setting with peers. Memory enhancement through cognitive stimulation and compensatory skill building are core elements in the programme. Other components include group problem solving, socialisation, peer support, exercise and camaraderie.

Outcomes

The Brookdale Foundation website does not provide information on research into the efficacy of the respite programmes or Early Memory Loss programmes they have funded.

Implementation

The Brookdale National Group Respite Program has stimulated a nationwide network of programmes providing regular activities, respite and support services for people with dementia and their carers. It declares that it has demonstrated that a cost-effective, social model of day services can successfully address the needs of people with dementia and their families. The Early Memory Loss programmes have also been offered across the US, in response to the growing population of earlier diagnosed people who seek resources to meet their special needs. To stimulate the dissemination the Brookdale Foundation has produced several guides on how to establish group activities and respite programmes for people with Alzheimer's disease and their families (Brookdale Foundation 1997), and how to plan and implement an Early Memory Loss programme (Einberger and Sellick 2006).[6]

---

6   See also www.brookdalefoundation.org

Conclusion

This chapter has described a range of support programmes for people with dementia and their carers living at home, most of which have developed rapidly in recent years. They aim to deliver timely support to people with dementia and carers, to promote their involvement and participation, and to create a continuum of support and care services starting after diagnosis and moving along the continuum of care. All programmes described are multicomponent, offering a variety of support such as information, communication, skills building, emotional support, participation and opportunities for social inclusion, albeit at different frequencies, intensity and at different stages of the disease.

The rapid and extensive spread of these programmes demonstrates the power of a socially driven model involving 'bottom-up' innovations to improve the opportunities for support offered to people with dementia and carers. The initiatives that focus on the social needs of people with dementia and their carers are highly appreciated and acceptable. This has the spin-off of motivating different organisations and agencies to contribute to the delivery of services and ultimately results in large numbers of people benefiting from social inclusion.

Another important aspect is the flexibility of these initiatives, particularly the Alzheimer Café, which allows for adaptation of the support to urban or rural areas, to different countries and cultures, or to differences in available resources, thus allowing support to be attuned to the different needs and contexts of individuals with dementia. Within the umbrella of Alzheimer Cafés, for example, a variety of initiatives are organised, differing in frequency and content, but what they all have in common are the café setting, regular meetings, continuity and the participation of the people with dementia during the café meetings.

A drawback of the Alzheimer Café initiatives, the Bistrot Mémoire and the Brookdale Foundation programmes, is the lack of substantive research on efficacy and efficiency. Their development can be seen as a modelling phase of an intervention, but further research is needed to better understand the specific outcomes as well as the factors related to their success. There are emerging studies that attempt to do this. For example a qualitative study of Alzheimer Cafés notes that despite the diversity of structure and activities, there were many similarities in family carer reports of their value (Greenwood *et al.* 2017). The Dutch MCSP is perhaps the most rigorously evaluated method and systematically translated across three other European nations (Brooker *et al.* 2017;

Mangiaracina *et al.* 2017; Szcześniak *et al.* 2018; Westerman *et al.* 2017) and practice dissemination (Brooker *et al.* 2017; 2018). The MEETINGDEM study also provides a framework for adapting the concept to particular country contexts, where stakeholders can become involved in developing the service to local requirements. Dissemination of MCSP across Europe and beyond is the next step for furthering research and practice into this type of innovation. Flexibility with adherence to the core concepts, systematic consideration of implementation strategies with relevant training, and ongoing monitoring will all be important ingredients in future spread of such programmes.

Learning from these initiatives can be situated on a continuum of intensity of support: at one end of the spectrum there are the Alzheimer Cafés and Memory Clubs, organised as monthly meetings in a community or public place, with the main objectives being to provide information, to meet peers and to discuss dementia-related issues for people with dementia and their carers; then the Bistrot Mémoire and Meeting Places where people come together in a café, restaurant or public space more often (once a week or fortnightly) and can participate in meaningful activities; and, at the other end of the spectrum, the more intensive Meeting Centres Support Programme and Brookdale respite programmes where day clubs are available several days a week and aspects of case management can be seen. These offer combined and separate support and social activities for people with dementia and carers. The DSCs in Austria provide stage-specific services and case management with ongoing monitoring and span the continuum for people with dementia and carers, across urban and rural areas.

References

Auer, S.R., Span, E. and Reisberg, B. (2015) 'Dementia Service Centres in Austria: A comprehensive support and early detection model for persons with dementia and their caregivers – theoretical foundations and model description.' *Dementia 14*, 4, 513–527.

Brookdale Foundation (1997) *How to Start and Manage Group Activities and Respite Programs for People with Alzheimer's Disease and Their Families: A Guide for Community-Based Organizations* (3rd edn). New York: The Brookdale Foundation.

Brooker, D., Dröes, R.M. and Evans, S. (2017) 'Framing outcomes of post-diagnostic psychosocial interventions in dementia: The Adaptation-Coping Model and adjusting to change.' *Working with Older People 21*, 1, 13–21.

Brooker, D., Evans, S., Evans, S., Bray, J. *et al.* (2018) 'Evaluation of the implementation of the Meeting Centres Support Program in Italy, Poland, and the UK; Exploration of the effects on people with dementia.' *International Journal of Geriatric Psychiatry 33*, 7, 883–892.

Capus, J. (2005) 'The Kingston dementia café: The benefits of establishing an Alzheimer café for carers and people with dementia.' *Dementia 4*, 588–591.

Coulon, P. and Sipos, I. (2013) 'Le dévelopment des Bistrots Mémoire en France.' *Neurologie-Psychiatrie-Geriatrie, 13*, 45–50. (In French)

Dow, B., Haralambous, B., Hempton, C., Hunt, S. and Calleja, D. (2011) 'Evaluation of Alzheimer's Australian Vic Memory Lane Cafés.' *International Psychogeriatrics 23*, 2, 246–255.

Dröes, R.M., Breebaart, E., Ettema, T.P., Van Tilburg, W. and Mellenbergh, G.J. (2000) 'The effect of integrated family support versus day care only on behaviour and mood of patients with dementia.' *International Psychogeriatrics 12*, 1, 99–116.

Dröes, R.M., Breebaart, E., Meiland, F.J.M., Van Tilburg, W. and Mellenbergh, G.J. (2004a) 'Effect of Meeting Centres Support Programme on feeling of competence of family caregivers and delay of institutionalization of people with dementia.' *Aging & Mental Health 8*, 3, 201–211.

Dröes, R.M., Meiland, F.J.M., Schmitz, M.J. and Van Tilburg, W. (2004b) 'Effect of combined support for people with dementia and carers versus regular day care on behaviour and mood of persons with dementia: Results from a multi-centre implementation study.' *International Journal of Geriatric Psychiatry 19*, 1–12.

Dröes, R.M., Meiland, F.J.M. and Van Tilburg, W. (2006a) 'The Meeting Centres Support Programme for Persons with Dementia and Their Carers: From Development to Implementation.' In B. Miesen and G. Jones (eds) *Caregiving in Dementia IV* (pp.315–339). London: Routledge.

Dröes, R.M., Meiland, F.J.M., Schmitz, M.J. and Van Tilburg, W. (2006b) 'Effect of the Meeting Centres Support Program on informal carers of people with dementia: Results from a multi-centre study.' *Aging & Mental Health 10*, 2, 112–124.

Dröes, R.M., Meiland, F.J.M., Schmitz, M. and Van Tilburg, W. (2011) 'An evaluation of the Meeting Centres Support Programme among persons with dementia and their carers.' *Nonpharmacological Therapies in Dementia 2*, 1, 19–39.

Dröes, RM. and Van Ganzewinkel, J. (2015) *Draaiboek Ontmoetingscentra voor mensen met dementie en hun verzorgers.* Amsterdam, 3ᵉ herziene druk. (In Dutch)

Dröes, R.M., Meiland, F. J. M., Evans, S., Brooker, D. *et al.* (2017) 'Comparison of the adaptive implementation and evaluation of the Meeting Centers Support Program for people with dementia and their family carers in Europe: Study protocol of the MEETINGDEM project.' *BMC Geriatrics 17*, 79, 1–12.

Einberger, K. and Sellick, J. (2006) *How to Plan and Implement an Early Memory Loss Program.* New York: The Brookdale Foundation.

Gaugler, J.E., Gallagher-Winker, K., Kehrberg, K., Lunde, A.M. *et al.* (2011) 'The memory club: Providing support to persons with early-stage dementia and their care partners.' *American Journal of Alzheimer's disease and Other Dementias 26*, 3, 218–226.

Greenwood, N., Smith, R., Akhtar, F. and Richardson, A. (2017) 'A qualitative study of carers' experiences of dementia cafés: A place to feel supported and be yourself.' *BMC Geriatrics 17*, 164.

Halley, E., Boulton, R., Mcfadzen, D. and Moriarty, J. (2005) 'The Poppy Café: A multi-agency approach to developing an Alzheimer café.' *Dementia 4*, 4, 592–594.

Logsdon, R.G., Pike, K.C., McCurry, S.M., Hunter, P. *et al.* (2010) 'Early-stage memory loss support groups: Outcomes from a randomized controlled clinical trial.' *Journals of Gerontology: Series B 65*, 6, 691–697.

Mangiaracina, F., Chattat, R., Farina, E., Saibene, F.L. *et al.* (2017) 'Not re-inventing the wheel: The adaptive implementation of the meeting centres support programme in four European countries.' *Aging & Mental Health, 21*, 1, 40–48.

Mather, L. (2006) 'Memory Lane Café: Follow-up support for people with early stage dementia and their families and carers.' *Dementia, 5,* 2, 290–293.

Mechtler, R. (2008) *Evaluation of the Dementia Service Centers in Upper Austria.* Evaluation Report (Institut für Pflege-und Gesundheitsforschung). Austria: Kepler University Linz. (In German)

Meiland, F.J., Dröes, R.M., De Lange, J. and Vernooij-Dassen, M.J. (2005) 'Facilitators and barriers in the implementation of the meeting centres model for people with dementia and their carers.' *Health Policy 7,* 2, 243–253.

Meiland, F.J.M., Dröes, R.M., De Lange, J., Vernooij-Dassen, M.J.F.J. and Van Tilburg, W. (2010) 'Predictors of effective support in meeting centers for people with dementia and their carers.' *Nonpharmacological Therapies in Dementia 1,* 3, 251–270.

Miesen, B. and Jones, G. (2004) 'The Alzheimer Café Concept: A Response to the Trauma, Drama and Tragedy of Dementia.' In G. Jones and B. Miesen (eds) *Care-giving in Dementia: Research and Applications. Vol. 3* (pp.307–333). London: Routledge.

Penna, A. (2012) *À quelle source doivent boire les Bistrots mémoire,* Nantes: le canard social. Accessed on 7/8/2017 at www.lecanardsocial.com/ArticleFil.aspx?i=795

Reisberg, B., Ferris, S., de Leon, M. and Crook, T. (1982) 'The Global Deterioration Scale for assessment of primary degenerative dementia.' *American Journal of Psychiatry 139,* 1136–1139.

Schultz, H., Auer, S., Span, E., Adler, C. *et al.* (2012) 'The educational model for M.A.S trainers.' *Zeitschrift für Gerontologie und Geriatrie 45,* 637–664. (In German)

Smits, C.H., de Lange, J., Dröes, R.M., Meiland, F., Vernooij-Dassen, M. and Pot, A.M. (2007) 'Effects of combined intervention programmes for people with dementia living at home and their caregivers: A systematic review.' *International Journal of Geriatric Psychiatry 22,* 1181–1193.

Szcześniak. D., Dröes, R.M., Meiland, F., Brooker, D. *et al.* (2018) 'Does the community-based combined Meeting Center Support Programme (MCSP) make the pathway to day-care activities easier for people living with dementia? A comparison before and after implementation of MCSP in three European countries.' *International Psychogeriatrics 30,* 11, 1717–1734.

Westerman, M.J., Farina, E., van der Sanden, M.C., Saibene, F.L. *et al.* (2017) 'Implementation of the Dutch Meeting Centres Support Program for people with dementia and their carers in Milan: Process evaluation of the preparation phase.' *Italian Society of Gerontology and Geriatrics 65,* 1–12.

Zarit, S.H., Femia, E.E., Watson, J., Rice-Oeschger, L. and Kakos, B. (2004) 'Memory club: A group intervention for people with early-stage dementia and their partners.' *The Gerontologist 44,* 2, 262–269.

Related reading

Evans, S., Evans, S., Brooker, D., Henderson, C. *et al.* (2018) 'The impact of the implementation of the Dutch combined Meeting Centres Support Programme for family caregivers of people with dementia in Italy, Poland and UK.' [Epub ahead of print.] *Aging & Mental Health.* doi:10.1080/13607863.2018.1544207

Jones, G.M.M. (2010) *The Alzheimer Café: Why It Works.* Sunninghill: The Wide Spectrum Ltd.

Mazurek, J., Szcześniak D, Malgorzata Lion, K., Dröes, R.M., Karczewski, M. and Rymaszewska (2019) 'Does the Meeting Centres Support Programme reduce unmet care needs of community-dwelling older people with dementia? A controlled, 6-month follow-up Polish Study.' *Clinical Interventions in Aging, 14,* 113–122.

For Emilia-Romagna Annual Plan: http://sociale.regione.emilia-romagna.it/anziani/temi/alzheimer-e-demenze-senili

For translation of MCSP: www.neurodegenerationresearch.eu/2016/10/meetingdem-progress-update-how-one-jpnd-project-is-bringing-a-tried-and-tested-dutch-model-for-dementia-care-to-italy-poland-and-the-uk

For the UK toolkit: www.worcester.ac.uk/about/academic-schools/school-of-allied-health-and-community/allied-health-research/association-for-dementia-studies/ads-research/uk-meeting-centres.aspx

Cognitive Stimulation Therapy (CST) for People with Dementia Living in the Community

Elisa Aguirre, Aimee Spector, Amy Streater and Martin Orrell

Introduction

Cognitive stimulation has been defined as engagement in a range of activities aimed at general enhancement of cognitive and social functioning, and is a distinct concept from cognitive rehabilitation and cognitive training (Clare and Woods 2004). Reality orientation (Woods 2002), conducted in hospitals as a form of mental therapy, is often seen as the precursor of cognitive stimulation therapy (CST). This chapter outlines: the development and evidence of group-based CST for people with dementia; principles of best practice including some of the factors to consider in running CST and longer term maintenance CST (mCST) groups; and experience of implementation into practice. Readers are signposted to international CST innovation in research and practice.

Overview: Development, evidence and practice of CST in the UK

CST was developed by combining effective elements from three Cochrane Reviews, of reality orientation, reminiscence therapy and validation therapy (Spector *et al.* 2000), to enhance both mental (cognitive) and social functioning. It was piloted as a group intervention (Spector *et al.* 2001) and then examined in a randomised controlled trial (RCT). This showed effectiveness for both cognition and quality of life outcomes and economic benefits (Knapp *et al.* 2006; Spector *et al.* 2003). Larger improvements in cognition were described as equivalent to the 'anti-dementia drugs' (i.e. the acetylcholinesterase inhibitors – AChEIs). Analysis of the cost of providing CST in England suggested that CST could generate a net benefit of nearly £54.9 million per year for the NHS (NHS 2011). An updated Cochrane Review of five RCTs and 718 people with dementia suggested that CST has a beneficial effect on memory and thinking; people who took part reported improved quality of life; and there were reported improvements in communication and interaction (Woods *et al.* 2012).

The first CST trial involved a seven-week programme of twice-weekly sessions with reported clinical and cost benefits. This led to the question of whether such changes could be maintained over a longer period, with a smaller 'dose', since two sessions per week were often not practical in the longer term. Therefore 'maintenance CST' (mCST), a 24-session programme designed to run once a week following completion of the initial CST programme, was developed. The pilot sessions followed similar themes and format to the CST programme (Aguirre *et al.* 2011a; Spector, Aguirre and Orrell 2010a), stakeholder feedback was taken (Aguirre *et al.* 2011b) and the CST manual was updated (Aguirre *et al.* 2011c). The RCT of mCST reported its cost-effectiveness (D'Amico *et al.* 2015) and effectiveness in improving quality of life and activities of daily living in people with dementia (Orrell *et al.* 2014). A sub-analysis of the data for people taking cholinesterase inhibitor medication showed that cognition in participants was better if they continued mCST (Orrell *et al.* 2014).

There are detailed manuals for those running CST groups (Aguirre *et al.* 2011c; Spector *et al.* 2006), but various versions of cognitive stimulation occur in practice, including differences in the duration and frequency of the programme offered. There is no clear relationship between dosage (length of the sessions x frequency x duration in weeks) and the effect size on cognitive function, or whether the frequency of sessions per week makes much of a difference (Woods *et al.* 2012). One study suggests that weekly CST does not offer the necessary 'dose' required to combat cognitive decline (Cove, Jacobi and Donovan 2014). In England, around two thirds of memory services for older people use group-CST but many may not adhere to the structured seven-week programme of two sessions per week; and services may use other measures of outcome – see for example an audit of effect of CST groups on 'mental wellbeing' (Allward *et al.* 2017).

Individualised CST (iCST) for people and their family carers at home has also been developed and tested. A trial demonstrated an enhanced quality of the caregiving relationship and improved quality of life for the carer (Orrell *et al.* 2017). The differences in key principles adopted for iCST compared with CST are outlined in Table 5.1 (see 'Further information' for details of the iCST manual).

The CST programme: CST and mCST

The CST programme includes 14 sessions, each lasting for 45–60 minutes. Owing to difficulties in getting the same group together twice a week, some services offer two sessions on the same day, with a break in between (which was also the case for some centres in the Spector *et al.* 2003 trial), whilst others may offer only once-weekly sessions. Each session ideally has two facilitators, and the same group of five to eight participants. Groups work best if participants have similar levels of cognitive ability, so that activities can be pitched accordingly. Each session begins with a warm-up activity (e.g. participants play catch with a soft ball and introduce themselves), designed to encourage group interaction and increase alertness. Participants then begin with some general orientation, including discussion of key news headlines. Next follows a main theme activity – consisting of stimulation exercises, grouped by theme (e.g. food, childhood, sounds, physical exercises, famous faces, word and number games).

Each CST session contains exercises of different types, focusing on memory, concentration, and linguistic and executive abilities. At the close of a session, participants are thanked for their contributions and participation; session ideas are summarised, and feedback is encouraged. The group's theme song, chosen along with the group's name at the outset of the programme, is sung at the opening and closing of each session. The group is reminded of the start time of the next session before they bid farewell.

The mCST programme comprises 24 weekly maintenance sessions based on the theoretical concepts of cognitive stimulation and grounded in the original CST programme. These maintenance sessions follow similar themes, but aim to use different materials wherever possible, as it is important that boredom is avoided for both members and facilitators.

Each session's structure is the same as that for the initial CST sessions. The mCST sessions were developed using a review of the evidence on cognitive stimulation and include additional themes that were not in the original CST programme. Professionals were consulted about the draft manual. These involved people with dementia, family carers and members of staff running activities for people with dementia. This led to further revision and the development of the second published CST manual (Aguirre *et al.* 2011c).

The structural framework of the CST sessions (with small groups of five to eight people) enables participants to meet others in similar situations, which in turn can serve to reduce their anxiety. The assumption is that when individuals gather together to share their concerns, they cope better with the potential stress of having dementia than they would on their own. The group allows:

- emotional bonding that creates closeness and reduces feelings of isolation

- enhanced self-esteem through sharing coping strategies

- information exchange to create a sense of hope and efficacy.

Key principles

Eighteen guiding principles are detailed in the mCST manual (Aguirre *et al.* 2011c). The first ten are specific to CST whereas the final eight are generic to any group dynamic intervention (Table 5.1). The aim is to enhance mental activity and engagement in different activities, which should also be enjoyable for people with dementia. Participants are always encouraged to develop new ideas, thoughts and associations. A good example of how to do this is in the 'faces' session. In typical group work, people might be shown a picture of a famous face and asked questions such as 'Who is this?' or 'What do you remember about them?'. However, in a CST session participants are shown two or more pictures at once and presented with questions such as 'What do these people have in common?', 'How are they different?', 'Who would you rather be?' and 'Who is more attractive to you?'. Similarly in the current affairs sessions, rather than introducing familiar topics (e.g. 'What do you think of the royal family?'), people are encouraged to discuss new topics, such as 'In your opinion is modern art really art?'

and 'What do you think of same sex weddings?'. Orientation is at the centre of the programme and is used sensitively and implicitly. Reality orientation (RO) and the rehearsal of orientation information (such as the date) can 'put people on the spot' with direct questions (e.g. 'What is your address?') that are seen as potentially demoralising. Therefore, orientation needs to be done in a subtle, implicit way at the beginning of each CST session. The date, name of group and group members, activity of the day and news headline are always written on the 'RO board', and facilitators of the programme refer to the board during the discussion. Participants are subtly orientated when introducing the session and discussing something in the news. For example, facilitators are encouraged to say 'Do you think this weather is typical for October, or do you find this weather hotter/colder than usual?' or 'Is anyone's birthday around now?' Also, many of the activities within themes provide scope for time orientation, for example by making a collage with autumn leaves in 'Being creative' or bringing in Christmas specialities for the 'Food' session.

The programme aims to create an environment where people have fun and learn, and where they strengthen their abilities and relationships amongst the group members, thus maintaining their social and cognitive skills at their optimum ability. CST aims to stimulate people via implicit rather than explicit learning, thus reducing the anxiety of feeling 'put on the spot'. The approach rests on asking people their opinions rather than searching for facts. This process often enables participants to recall names later without the need for explicit questions. CST focuses on a variety of individually tailored, multisensory stimulation exercises (e.g. matching common sounds to pictures in the 'Sounds' session). People are involved in decision-making and encouraged to interact among themselves, rather than just with the group facilitator. Reminiscence is integrated as a means of orientation in the programme, for example through the comparison of old and new coins, prices and objects, and the discussion of current affairs (e.g. the war in Syria in comparison with memories of the Second World War).

The RO board is a useful way of triggering memories and aiding recall. Multisensory cues are an essential aspect of the programme, and memory and learning are supported in the intervention through providing continuity and consistency between sessions. Examples of this include referring to the group name, always running the group in the same room, and starting sessions and ending sessions in a similar way (e.g. using a warm-up and singing songs). Many of the sessions stimulate language, for example naming of people and objects (e.g. in categorisation), thinking about word construction and word association, which may be why language skills appear to improve following CST (Spector, Orrell and Woods 2010b). Executive functioning skills are also stimulated in the intervention, especially involving planning and organising, for example, planning and executing stages of a task (such as making a cake) in 'Being creative'. Mental organisation is exercised through the discussion of similarities and differences in several sessions, word association and categorising objects.

Table 5.1: CST key principles (* denotes iCST key principles)

1	Mental stimulation
2	New ideas, thoughts and associations
3	Using orientation, sensitively and implicitly
4	Opinions, rather than facts*
5	Using reminiscence, and as an aid to the here and now*
6	Providing triggers to aide recall*
7	Continuity and consistency between sessions
8	Implicit (rather than explicit) learning
9	Stimulating language*
10	Stimulating executive functioning
11	Person-centred*
12	Respect
13	Involvement
14	Inclusion
15	Choice* in home-based CST activities
16	Fun* enjoyment and fun for person and carer
17	Maximising potential*
18	Building strengthening relationships* [strengthening the caregiving relationship]

CST theory – how it might work for people with dementia?

Dementia is a condition that has some fixed factors that are less likely to be amenable to change and tractable factors that are more amenable to change (Spector and Orrell 2010c). CST provides a means for mental and personalised social stimulation in a stable environment.

Mental stimulation

Dementia is characterised by declining cognition, but people with dementia can have reserve capacity for cognitive information-processing. Implicit memory in Alzheimer's disease is preserved for a longer period than episodic memory and responds to regular stimulation (Fleischman, Wilson and Gabrieli 2005). Multisensory and mental stimulation (such as imagery, categorical classification and semantic association) aims to maximise episodic and semantic memory functions and consolidate implicit memory. Beneficial effects on cognition may involve both implicit and residual explicit memory (Tailby and Haslam 2003). Therefore CST provides global stimulation of cognitive abilities: memory, concentration, language, executive functioning, spatio-temporal orientation and visuo-constructive abilities, with particular benefits in promoting language and generating opinions, and with potential to create new semantic links through categorisation and associated generalised cognitive outcomes (Spector et al. 2010b).

An important element in CST is stimulation of orientation. Each session includes an orientation board, enabling participants to discuss current information and news. Another element of the programme is the use of physical activity in the sessions, including ten minutes of warm-up activity at the beginning of each session, and a session theme called 'Physical games'. This is an important element for frail people who have little movement as it offers an element of physical activity.

Personalised social stimulation

CST activities are set in a social context where both group engagement and personalised activities are important. The in-session activities have flexibility to adapt to participant interests and abilities. Each theme contains exercises of different types, including categorical classifications, old/new comparisons of objects, numerical and musical exercises designed to enrich the general cognitive experience and use of implicit strategies for word and concept recall. The latter is important for increasing confidence, lost through cognitive problems and the consequent anxiety of forgetting words in the middle of a conversation that may lead to social withdrawal. CST uses reminiscence as an aid to orientation; this may contribute to the psychological health of people with dementia given that the progressive deteriorating nature of the disease erodes the ability to succeed in a range of previous enjoyable activities. People with dementia may retain the capacity to recall and integrate the past through spared remote memory through most of the dementia process.

A possible mechanism for quality of life change is that the CST approach is grounded in a strong value base of respecting individuality and personhood within a social setting. The different CST principles serve as strategies to fulfil the needs of identity, attachment, comfort, inclusion, occupation and love, outlined by Kitwood (1997).

The CST approach to person-centred care incorporates:

- *Biographical knowledge of the person.* This helps facilitators to adapt the different sessions according to the individual's needs and interest. The use of reminiscence to promote person-centred practice acts as an aid to the here and now. It is thought to affirm the experiences and views of the world of people with dementia and foster social interaction through sharing of autobiographical memories using multisensory stimuli such as pictures, music and scrapbooks.

- *A focus on opinion rather than facts.* This acknowledges the person's interpretation of reality through validation of their individual experiences. This unconditional positive regard may promote confidence and wellbeing. CST sessions offer freedom of expression and a release from previous constraints and concerns, to present new sources of pleasure and satisfaction for the person with dementia.

- *Person-centredness.* This incorporates valuing every person in the group and helping them to feel content; offering opportunities for dignity and striving to preserve a sense of self; accepting each person's 'way of being' and opinions; sharing everyday life with a sense of togetherness (ten minutes included before the session with refreshments for extra social interaction); encouraging a sense of belonging to the group (selecting their group name and song in the first session of the programme); offering a secure environment (consistency of environment throughout the programme); providing opportunities for occupation through the different proposed activities; and promoting a sense of power and control (encouraging different participant roles within the group).

Environment

The setting for the CST groups and the consistency of environment ('a sense of place') between sessions, (e.g. using the same place and session structure) promotes comfort and stability at a time of great uncertainty for people with dementia, who can become isolated due to their condition. Small groups are used to promote social interaction and relationships.

Implementation of CST

Implementation involves looking at an intervention and its applicability in a real-life setting. The CST programme was designed to be delivered by any health or care professional with experience of working with people with dementia, and it can be conducted in a variety of settings. One-day in-house CST facilitator training events are available in the UK[1] and many centres have now started running local CST groups.[2] A training manual for group facilitators can be purchased from Hawker Publications[3] (Aguirre et al. 2011c; Spector et al. 2006). Manuals include a list of equipment needed for running the CST and maintenance CST programmes along with other relevant resources.

Training and implementation research

Spector, Orrell and Aguirre (2011) asked 76 practitioners who had attended one-day CST training whether they had subsequently set up CST groups and encountered any obstacles. Better learning characteristics among those who had been trained demonstrated a likeliness to take up CST, while factors such as lack of time and resources proved a barrier to setting up a CST programme. All 27 people who

---

1   See www.cstdementia.com/page/training-and-events
2   See www.cstdementia.com
3   www.hawkerpublications.co.uk

reported that they had run CST groups said they had encountered some difficulties: 11 (41%) highlighted a lack of staff time, six (23%) a lack of resources, four (15%) not enough suitable participants, two (7%) no suitable room, two (7%) transport problems, and two (7%) lack of support from management. For those 49 people who did not run CST groups, reasons were: lack of staff time (44%), lack of resources (14%), no suitable room (11%), not enough suitable participants (11%), transport problems (10%), not feeling skilled enough (7%), and lack of support from management (3%). So, although 93 per cent reported feeling adequately skilled following a training day, this was not enough to put CST into practice everywhere. Factors to improve implementation of CST included: wanting more support from other staff members, regular supervision from a specialist, an online forum, training in other areas, and regular supervision. This feedback enabled further development of the CST programme to determine whether such additional support might influence the implementation and uptake of CST.

A multi-centre, pragmatic RCT with 241 staff members working in a variety of care settings was carried out comparing the effectiveness of outreach support versus no outreach support when delivering CST and mCST in practice (Streater *et al.* 2012). The researchers hypothesised that the average number of attendees would differ between the two groups, but no difference was found (Streater *et al.* 2017). In addition, no difference was found in staff outcomes. A separate study however, found that care home staff who received training and ongoing support significantly improved in positive approaches to dementia care and sense of competence (Streater *et al.* 2016a). An observational study of 89 people with dementia was conducted to determine whether positive outcomes associated with CST and mCST, specifically cognition and quality of life, could be demonstrated in practice (Streater *et al.* 2016b). When the authors controlled for mild to moderate level of cognition using the Mini Mental State Examination (MMSE: Folstein, Folstein and McHugh 1975), a significant improvement in cognition was demonstrated whilst quality of life remained unchanged.

Key features required for implementation in routine practice

Setting up a local CST group

In preparing for a CST group, we recommend that potential participants are screened initially, in order to identify their strengths, sensitivities and interests. Two assessment tools have been identified as useful for practical CST group progress evaluations: the MMSE (Folstein *et al.* 1975) for measuring cognition, and QoL-AD (Logsdon *et al.* 2002) for measuring quality of life. Assessing participants using these two tools can also give an indication of positive changes in cognition and quality of life following attendance. Due to copyright charges for the MMSE, many people now use the Montreal Cognitive Assessment[4] or the ACE-R[5] in clinical practice.

The feedback gathered from participants attending local groups has been very positive. Participants have reported enjoying the groups, feeling pleasure in sharing their experiences, and valuing the chance to offer help and advice to others. They also express appreciation for the chance to develop and relearn skills that have helped them to work with their illness as reflected in the quotes from participants in a CST group (see box below).

Comments from CST programme participants (from Knowles 2010)

'I can relax. The use of the visual aids helps think things through, we share the same problem, and all like coming, otherwise, we wouldn't be here.'

'Over the time I noticed everyone becoming more relaxed and not having to be worried if you say the wrong thing'.

'We just enjoy ourselves, there's an awful lot of laughing.'

'You feel like a little family.'

Qualitative interviews and focus groups with people with dementia attending CST groups, their carers and the group facilitators (Spector, Gardner and Orrell 2011) describe two emerging themes 'Positive

---

4   www.mocatest.org
5   www.acer.org

experiences of being in the group' and 'Changes experienced in everyday life'. The overall experience of attending CST was seen as being emotionally positive, and most participants reported some cognitive benefits. There were reports, for example, of feeling more positive, relaxed and confident within themselves, as well as specific improvements in memory, concentration and alertness (Spector *et al.* 2011).

Overcoming practical obstacles to running CST

There may be logistical difficulties in planning and arranging groups in settings where participants need to be escorted to the group, or transport needs to be organised. Other potential problems have been reported when trying to engage people with dementia with a wide range of cognitive abilities, in a therapeutic group activity. It can be hard to pitch the activities at a level to suit the whole group. Thus, some group members may become frustrated with more cognitively impaired group members, who may subsequently feel very aware of their losses. However, careful, skilled structuring and adequate staffing to overcome these types of obstacles during a group session can resolve these problems – see Brooker and Duce (2000) for guidance on group work in dementia services.

International perspectives

Guidelines to adapting group-CST to cultural needs have been published (Aguirre, Spector and Orrell 2014; Aguirre and Werheid 2018). CST remains flourishing as a research and practice innovation internationally. Practice manuals and published efficacy studies can be found in many countries.[6]

Conclusion

CST for dementia is now well established in the UK as a frontline therapy for people with mild to moderate dementia, which should be available regardless of whether or not people receive 'anti-dementia' medication. For example, it remains a recommended therapy within the recently updated NICE guidance, where services are advised to 'Offer group cognitive stimulation therapy to people living with mild

---

6   See www.ucl.ac.uk/international-cognitive-stimulation-therapy for country-specific knowledge and tools; Yates *et al.* 2017.

to moderate dementia' (NICE 2018). A Cochrane Review (Woods *et al.* 2012) and other research confirm the short- and medium-term benefits of CST, and economic analyses suggest it could save the NHS money. Group-CST is now available in two thirds of UK memory services, although the 'dosage' (number of sessions) may vary. At the time of writing, group-CST can be found in 23 countries worldwide.[7]

References

Aguirre, E., Spector, A., Hoe, J., Streater, A. *et al.* (2011a) 'Development of an evidence-based extended programme of maintenance cognitive stimulation therapy (CST) for people with dementia. *Non-pharmacological Therapies in Dementia 1*, 3, 198–215.

Aguirre, E., Spector, A., Streater, A., Burnell, K. and Orrell, M. (2011b) 'Service users' involvement in the development of a maintenance cognitive stimulation therapy (CST) programme: A comparison of the views of people with dementia, staff and family carers.' *Dementia 10*, 4, 459–473.

Aguirre, E., Spector, A., Streater, A., Hoe, J., Woods, B. and Orrell, M. (2011c) *Making a Difference 2. An Evidence-Based Group Programme to Offer Maintenance Cognitive Stimulation Therapy (CST) to People with Dementia.* London: Hawker Publications.

Aguirre, E., Spector, A. and Orrell, M. (2014) 'Guidelines to adapt cognitive stimulation therapy (CST) to other cultures.' *Clinical Interventions in Aging 26*, 9, 1003–1007.

Aguirre, E. and Werheid, K. (2018) 'Guidelines for Adapting Cognitive Stimulation Therapy (CST) to Other Cultures.' In L.A. Yates *et al.* (eds) *Cognitive Stimulation Therapy for Dementia: History, Evolution and Internationalism* (pp.177–193). Abingdon: Routledge.

Allward, C., Dunn, R., Forshaw, G., Rewston, C. and Wass, N. (2017) 'Mental wellbeing in people with dementia following cognitive stimulation therapy.' [Epub ahead of print.] *Dementia.* doi:10.1177/1471301217722443.

Brooker, D. and Duce, L. (2000) 'Wellbeing and activity in dementia: A comparison of group reminiscence therapy, structured goal-directed group activity and unstructured time.' *Aging & Mental Health 4*, 4, 354–358.

Clare, L. and Woods, R.T. (2004) 'Cognitive training and cognitive rehabilitation for people with early-stage Alzheimer's disease: A review.' *Neuropsychological Rehabilitation 14*, 385–401.

Cove, J., Jacobi, N. and Donovan, H. (2014) 'Effectiveness of weekly cognitive stimulation therapy for people with dementia and the additional impact of enhancing cognitive stimulation therapy with a carer training program.' *Clinical Interventions in Aging 11*, 9, 2143–2150.

D'Amico, F., Rehill, A., Knapp, M., Aguirre, E. *et al.* (2015) 'Maintenance cognitive stimulation therapy: An economic evaluation within a randomised controlled trial.' *Journal of the American Medical Directors Association (JAMDA) 16*, 1, 63–70.

Fleischman, D.A., Wilson, R.S. and Gabrieli, J.D. (2005) 'Implicit memory and Alzheimer's disease neuropathology.' *Brain 128*, 2006–2015.

Folstein, M.F., Folstein, S.E. and McHugh, P.R. (1975) 'Mini-mental state: A practical method for grading the cognitive state of patients for the clinician.' *Journal of Psychiatric Research 12*, 189–198.

---

7   See www.cstdementia.com

Kitwood, T. (1997) *Dementia Reconsidered: The Person Comes First.* Buckingham: Open University Press.

Knapp, M., Thorgrimsen, L., Patel, A., Spector, A. *et al.* (2006) 'Cognitive stimulation therapy for people with dementia: Cost-effectiveness analysis.' *British Journal of Psychiatry 188,* 6, 574–580.

Knowles, J. (2010) 'Early and better diagnosis for people with dementia – then what?' *Signpost: Journal of Dementia and Mental Health Care of Older People 14,* 3.

Logsdon, R.G., Gibbons, L.E., McCurry, S.M. and Teri, L. (2002) 'Assessing quality of life in older adults with cognitive impairment.' *Psychosomatic Medicine 64,* 510–519.

NHS Institute for Innovation and Improvement (2011) *An Economic Evaluation of Alternatives to Antipsychotic Drugs for Individuals Living with Dementia.* NHS Institute for Innovation and Improvement, University of Warwick Campus, Coventry.

NICE (National Institute for Health and Care Excellence) (2018) *Dementia – Assessment, Management and Support for People Living with Dementia and Their Carers.* NICE Clinical Guideline NG97. Accessed on 3/8/2018 at www.nice.org.uk/guidance/ng97

Orrell, M., Aguirre, E., Spector, A., Hoare, Z. *et al.* (2014) 'Maintenance cognitive stimulation therapy for dementia: Single-blind, multicentre, pragmatic randomised controlled trial.' *British Journal of Psychiatry 204,* 6, 454–461.

Orrell, M., Yates, L., Leung, P., Hoare, Z. *et al.* (2017) 'The impact of individual cognitive stimulation therapy (iCST) on cognition, quality of life, caregiver health, and family relationships in dementia: A randomized controlled trial.' *PloS Medicine 14,* 3, e1002269.

Spector, A., Davies, S., Woods, B. and Orrell, M. (2000) 'Reality orientation for dementia: A systematic review of the evidence of effectiveness from randomised controlled trials.' *The Gerontologist 40,* 206–212.

Spector, A., Orrell, M., Davies, S. and Woods, B. (2001) 'Can reality orientation be rehabilitated? Development and piloting of an evidence-based programme of cognition-based therapies for people with dementia.' *Neuropsychological Rehabilitation 11,* 3–4, 377–397.

Spector, A., Thorgrimsen, L., Woods, B., Royan, L. *et al.* (2003) 'Efficacy of an evidence based cognitive stimulation therapy programme for people with dementia: Randomised controlled trial.' *British Journal of Psychiatry 183,* 248–254.

Spector, A., Thorgrimsen, L., Woods, R.T. and Orrell, M. (2006) *Making a Difference.* London: Hawker Publications.

Spector, A., Aguirre, E. and Orrell, M. (2010a) 'Translating research into practice: A pilot study examining the use of cognitive stimulation therapy (CST) after a one-day training course.' *Non-pharmacological Therapies in Dementia 1,* 1, 61–70.

Spector, A., Orrell, M. and Woods, B. (2010b) 'Cognitive stimulation therapy (CST): Effects on different areas of cognitive function for people with dementia.' *International Journal of Geriatric Psychiatry 25,* 12, 1253–1258.

Spector, A. and Orrell, M. (2010c) 'Using a biopsychosocial model of dementia as a tool to guide clinical practice.' *International Psychogeriatrics 22,* 6, 957–965.

Spector, A., Gardner, C. and Orrell, M. (2011) 'The impact of cognitive stimulation therapy groups on people with dementia: Views from participants, their carers and group facilitators.' *Aging & Mental Health 15,* 8, 945–949.

Streater, A., Spector, A., Aguirre, E., Hoe, J. *et al.* (2012) 'Maintenance cognitive stimulation therapy (CST) in practice: Study protocol for a randomized controlled trial.' *Trials 13,* 91.

Streater, A. Aguirre, E. Spector, A. and Orrell, M. (2016a) 'Cognitive stimulation therapy for people with dementia in practice: A service evaluation.' *British Journal of Occupational Therapy 79,* 9, 574–580.

Streater, A., Spector, A., Aguirre, E. and Orrell, M. (2016b) 'Cognitive stimulation therapy (CST) for people with dementia in practice: An observational study.' *British Journal of Occupational Therapy 79*, 12, 762–767.

Streater, A., Spector, A., Aguirre, E. and Orrell, M. (2017) 'Staff training and outreach support for cognitive stimulation therapy (CST) and its implementation in practice: A cluster randomised trial.' *International Journal of Geriatric Psychiatry 32*, 12, e64–e71.

Tailby, R. and Haslam, C. (2003) 'An investigation of errorless learning in memory-impaired patients: Improving the technique and clarifying theory.' *Neuropsychologia 4*, 9, 1230–1240.

Woods R.T. (2002) 'Reality orientation: A welcome return?' *Age & Ageing 31*, 155–156.

Woods, B., Aguirre, E., Spector, A. and Orrell, M. (2012) 'Cognitive stimulation to improve cognitive functioning in people with dementia.' *Cochrane Database of Systematic Reviews*, Issue 2. Art. no. CD005562.

Yates, L. A., Yates, J., Orrell, M., Spector, A. and Woods, B. (eds) (2017) *Cognitive Stimulation Therapy for Dementia: History, Evolution and Internationalism.* Abingdon: Routledge.

Further information

Websites

For full details of cognitive stimulation therapy: www.cstdementia.com

CST worldwide with country-specific details: www.ucl.ac.uk/ international-cognitive-stimulation-therapy

Manuals

CST manuals, including iCST, available from www.hawkerpublications. co.uk

Chinese translation: Hong Kong University Press – contact Dr Gloria Wong Associate Professor: ghywong@hku.hk

German translation of Spector *et al.* 2006: *Kognitive Anregung (CST) für Menschen mit Demenz: Evidenzbasiertes Praxis- und Gruppenhandbuch* (2013, Huber).

International contexts

Capotosto, E., Belacchi, C., Gardini, S., Faggian, S. *et al.* (2016) 'Cognitive stimulation therapy in the Italian context: Its efficacy in cognitive and non-cognitive measures in older adults with dementia.' *International Journal of Geriatric Psychiatry 32*, 3, 331–340.

Mkenda, S., Olakehinde, O., Mbowe, G., Siwoku, A. *et al.* (2016) 'Cognitive stimulation therapy as a low-resource intervention for dementia in sub-Saharan Africa (CST-SSA): Adaptation for rural Tanzania and Nigeria.' *Dementia 7*, 4, 515–530.

Wong, G.H.Y., Yek, O.P.L., Zhang, A.Y., Lum, T.Y.S. and Spector, A. (2018) 'Cultural adaptation of cognitive stimulation therapy (CST) for Chinese people with dementia: Multicentre pilot study.' *International Journal of Geriatric Psychiatry 33*, 6, 841–848.

Yamanaka, K., Kawano, Y., Noguchi, D., Nakaaki, S. *et al.* (2013) 'Effects of cognitive stimulation therapy Japanese version (CST-J) for people with dementia: A single blind, controlled clinical trial.' *Aging & Mental Health, 17*, 5, 579–586.

Chapter 6

Promoting Participation in Meaningful Occupation

Gail Mountain and Sarah Kate Smith

Introduction

Over recent years, there has been growing interest in how people with dementia can be supported to manage the consequences of their condition and experience a good quality of life (sometimes referred to as self-management), and how family carers can be assisted to support the person to retain independence and self-efficacy for as long as possible. Through consultation with people with dementia and family carers Mountain and Craig (2012) identified priorities for self-management in dementia. Findings from the consultation confirmed the prime importance of retaining a good quality of life and continuing to experience life satisfaction while living with the diagnosis. Satisfaction can be achieved through continuing to undertake activities of daily living independently. However in common with the overall population, participation in social, leisure and recreational activities is highly likely to be enjoyable and contribute towards quality of life for people living with dementia. Significantly, individuals involved in the consultation articulated the importance of retaining involvement in aspects of life that did not remind them constantly of their diagnosis, such as assisting others in a voluntary capacity.

The validity of these consultation findings is confirmed by others' research. Continued participation can retain the personhood of the individual and their ability to relate to others (Phinney 2006). It can also decrease the risk of the individual becoming social isolated, and provide the tools that can assist to cope with some of the changes that accompany a diagnosis (Genoe 2013). Wang, Xu and Pei (2012) examined the current body of evidence and concluded that such participation also has a protective effect in helping to retain cognitive function. However, despite the importance of social and leisure interests and pastimes for mental, physical and cognitive wellbeing, participation in enjoyable activities is one of the most frequently identified unmet needs reported by people with dementia living in the community (Smits *et al.* 2007). Many people in the early stages of the condition are bored and sit at home with nothing to do even though ability to participate in enjoyable activities is retained (Phinney 2006). One explanation is that dementia lessens the ability to create one's own enjoyable activities (Topo 2008). Diminished interaction with others is a further 'social causality' arising from the condition, which leads to social isolation, relationship changes and loss of independence. It is unsurprising then that those with dementia are more likely than the general population to be depressed.

This chapter describes the value of continued engagement in social and leisure activities by people following a diagnosis of dementia who live in the community; and provides recommendations for the types of activities that can be beneficial and identifies how engagement can be encouraged and sustained. We propose that to avoid mental ill health, help to make life worth living and help to maintain abilities for as long as possible, people with dementia are entitled to have continued access to activities and opportunities for participation. Such activities are defined as being free time away from domestic chores and chosen by, rather than for, the person. They do not include the therapeutic activities that can be characteristic of day and residential care settings. They might be sedentary such as reading a book or completing a crossword, or active, for example going for a walk or playing golf, and can include volunteering and other forms of citizenship, social pastimes or individual hobbies depending upon personal choice.

Context

People with dementia used to be understood in terms of what they could no longer achieve (Sabat 2001), even though individuals who have the diagnosis are likely to focus upon the abilities that remain intact and adopt strategies to preserve their dignity (Sørensen, Waldorff and Waldemar 2008). Those with a diagnosis consistently report that their attitudes, beliefs, opinions and preferences are the same as they always were, despite dementia, and it is the symptoms and the reactions of others to their diagnosis and symptoms that makes them feel different (Sabat 2001). It is heartening that recent improvements in societal awareness and in dementia services are leading to an appreciation of the need to work with and build upon retained skills rather than solely focusing upon deficits. There is now a significant move to try and ensure the social inclusion of people with dementia, with enhanced participation being one means of achieving this.

This awareness has extended to the research environment where until recently, people with dementia have remained largely excluded from the research process, possibly due to the stigma associated with cognitive decline (Hellström *et al.* 2007). Rather, researchers have relied on 'proxy' accounts provided by the person's spouse or family member. This is problematic for two reasons. First, the perspectives and opinions of the person with dementia do not consistently correspond with their family carer. Second, there is a danger that the needs and requirements of the person with a diagnosis may be overlooked in favour of the family carer rendering the individual powerless and sidelined (Mountain and Craig 2012). This damage to the person's self-esteem can have important consequences for social relationships, new learning and overall wellbeing (Kitwood 1997), which may lead to assumptions regarding decreased interest and ability to participate effectively in society. However, there is increasing evidence to suggest that people in the earlier stages of the condition can be as fully aware as their family caregiver of their diagnosis and its immediate and future impact (Whitlatch *et al.* 2006). Topics of 'inclusion' have witnessed a shift in research to topics of 'participation'. This is important as the concept of 'inclusion' could imply that the individual with dementia is a passive addition to the process when reaching decisions about their lives, rather than actively participating in decisions because their opinions and perspectives matter (Bartlett and Connor 2007). The Dementia Care Advocacy and Support Network International (DASNI) is a clear example of advocacy communities that promote 'participation' as a fundamental right for everyone, irrespective of the stage of dementia.

It is not surprising that preferences for social and leisure activities by people with dementia are consistent with those of the older population in general and are highly heterogeneous irrespective of the stage of the condition (Menne *et al.* 2012). Moreover, leisure can become more significant to people following diagnosis with many individuals being keen to stay socially connected and engage in activities that are meaningful to them. People with dementia can be challenged in communicating their preferences, but interested if an activity is initiated by others. Sometimes the person will wish to continue to pursue long-standing interests, but, alternatively, insight into lessening abilities and/or changing interests may discourage the continuation of pastimes that were previously enjoyed. The fact that so many people living with dementia in their own homes are struggling to find something enjoyable and meaningful to do suggests that urgent support is needed to maintain participation in social and leisure activity.

Involving the family carer

Two thirds of people with dementia in the UK live in their own homes. This is the preference for the majority, and is also important as the familiarity of home can take on significant meaning, compensating for reductions in physical and mental functioning associated with dementia (Phinney 2006). The term *carer* is used to refer to those providing assistance in an unpaid capacity. Recent evidence from a meta-analysis suggests that psychosocial interventions that have been tailored to the person with dementia and their carer can be effective in two distinct ways. First, such engagement can promote wellbeing in the person with dementia and reduce psychological symptoms. Second, involvement can reduce carer burden and stress (Brodaty and Arasaratnam 2012). Nevertheless, the interests and needs of the person and their family carer will not always correspond and they will each have very different and sometimes inconsistent experiences of the dementia (Beard *et al.* 2012).

As the illness progresses, supporting involvement in such activities can be time-consuming and require imagination and creativity on the part of the family carer, who may be overwhelmed by everyday tasks (Nygård 2004). The challenge, therefore, is to determine how unmet needs for leisure might be met without placing undue demands upon the family carer. Attention is also required when matching the requirements of the person with dementia and their carer to a proposed activity, including how activities can be personalised to correspond with individual and dyadic preferences as well as optimum modes of delivery (Van't Leven *et al.* 2013). This confirms the need to identify a balance between the needs of the individual with dementia and the needs of the family carer without compromising the relationship between the two (Mountain and Craig 2012). Phinney (2006) identified three strategies used by family carers to support the person they care for with activity: first, structuring activities in such a way that reduces the demands on the person thus diminishing the impact of the condition; second, by guiding the person through the activity with use of instructions and reminders; third, by accompanying the person during the chosen activity. While these strategies may not be appropriate in all situations, this illustrates the value of enabling the family carer with clear and personalised advice and strategies to achieve and sustain necessary levels of support for anything beyond routine care.

Maintaining and developing opportunities for socialisation

Socialisation can be a central component of leisure activity, and in a study by Sørensen *et al.* (2008) a small number of people with early-stage dementia were asked to describe their experiences in everyday life, including any changes in activities and social life with family and friends. Some of those who participated described how they had begun to feel uncomfortable around others in case they might say something embarrassing, and others talked about how friends had stopped calling, resulting in fewer opportunities to remain socially connected. The study found that support from the family carer helped to maintain connections and decrease isolation, confirming the importance of family carers in maintaining social connectivity and diminishing the negative impact of dementia. This both emphasises the essential contribution of family carers but also questions how to fill the void if the person does not have a carer, or the carers are not able to facilitate continued social participation for whatever reason.

Nevertheless, activities that incorporate interactions with others, including face-to-face, telephone or through information and communication technology (ICT) may help to maintain positive interactions and subsequently promote a positive self-image. The ever increasing potential of internet-based social networking, including Skype, FaceTime, Facebook and blogging are already being harnessed to benefit communities of people with dementia and will likely develop and extend over time. These tools to maintain socialisation should be encouraged and supported irrespective of carer involvement. Further, these tools empower and give 'voice' as well as offering alternative ways to communicate leading to increased positive experiences (Clare, Rowlands and Quin 2008).

Meeting personal preferences

Persistent stereotypes can assume that people with dementia are only capable of participating in limited activity, yet, when they have been asked, wide variations of personal preference have been found. A survey by Menne *et al.* (2012) involved asking people with dementia about their preferences for social and leisure activities. Results identified socialising, TV music and radio, exercise and recreation, and activities for cognitive stimulation such as crosswords. Participants revealed that they were aware of the deficits associated with dementia and the ways in which the condition was affecting them could lead to perceptions of being undervalued by those closest to them. In order to preserve their dignity and feelings of self-worth individuals attempted to adjust their usual activities in ways that could conceal the difficulties they were experiencing. Menne *et al.* (2012) emphasised the importance of encouraging activities that the person finds enjoyable and the value of activity modification to compensate for cognitive decline; for example using audio rather than traditional books.

Having access to relevant information

Having access to high-quality information about the dementia syndrome is essential for both the person and their family carer post-diagnosis, so that they are able to understand the condition and use this knowledge to identify and adopt new ways of approaching life. As well as providing details of what to expect and how to self-manage the symptoms, information should also include details of local resources that might be able to help and/or provide outlets for participation and leisure. For example, Reid, Warnes and Low (2013) compiled the Sheffield Dementia Information Pack as a resource to support people living with memory problems. It is important that such information is not necessarily dementia-specific and incorporates resources that are mainstream and willing to provide the necessary assistance. Maintaining an up-to-date record is of prime importance so that the person with dementia and their carer can be confident in the accuracy of the information and avoid abortive journeys, which can be very damaging for individuals with already compromised personal resources.

Potential activities

As previously described, the personal preference for activity may range considerably from person to person and brief descriptions of some potential activities are now discussed.

Citizenship and volunteering

In the consultation described by Mountain and Craig (2012), participants described the benefits of engaging in 'normal' activities that also provide some form of contribution, such as assisting with the care of family pets and volunteering in local charity shops. Awareness of the benefits of engagement in such activities has led to some experimentation with programmes for people with dementia that incorporate real rather than contrived contributions but are also sympathetic to the needs of the volunteers.

Kinney, Kart and Reddecliff (2011) evaluated a very small-scale zoo volunteer programme for people with early-stage dementia. Results indicated benefits, not only for the individuals who participated but also for their extended family and for the wider community. The positive reactions of others bestowed status upon the participants. Identified limitations included the relatively high cost of the intervention and the focus upon providing such opportunities for those with early-onset dementia only. Another example of enabling people to continue active participation in volunteering activities involved gardening, with this project also illustrating a similar range of benefits but with high costs for few numbers (Hewitt et al. 2013).

Bruin et al. (2009) conducted research into 'green farms' in The Netherlands. This initiative is different from those recounted by Kinney et al. (2011) and Hewitt et al. (2013) and unique in that it was established as a viable alternative to day care. This concept has been promulgated beyond demonstration projects; the evaluation involved 11 such facilities for people in the moderate stages of the condition. Nevertheless, the principles of providing meaningful activity were the same, as were the benefits that participants derived from engagement in structured outdoor physical activity. Results indicated that individuals were involved in activities most (75%) of the time compared with just over half (55%) at the regular daycare facility. The authors consider the increase of individual involvement at the green farms to be due to a more stimulating and activating environment, thus creating ample opportunity to be involved in a variety of activities.

Physical activity

Exercise is important for everyone and in common with the overall population people with dementia can derive tangible benefits from regular physical activity, as illustrated by the previous examples of involvement in gardening and farms. Gains include maintenance of functional abilities and improved sleep patterns with higher intensity activities leading to greater benefits (Potter *et al.* 2011). For some people, dementia can manifest in a tendency to wander, and there is weak evidence to suggest that this can be allayed by appropriate exercise (Robinson *et al.* 2007), with the authors also observing that the literature is limited by the lack of engagement of people with dementia in choices of activity. Physical exercise can be combined with a pleasurable activity, such as walking; there is a small evidence base to suggest that people with dementia find 'green exercise' such as walking in the countryside enjoyable, but once again this evidence is commensurate with that concerning the older population overall.

Engagement in new technologies

In common with the overall population, people with dementia are able to enjoy technologies for leisure and recreation. The greater accessibility of new forms of touch screen and tablet devices is increasing possibilities beyond the old stereotypical interpretation of technology for people with dementia, which is focused upon safety, security and providing carer reassurance. However, this move to assist people with dementia to benefit from the leisure opportunities offered by technologies in similar ways to that of the general population is only just commencing, and there is little published research in this area.

A project convened by the University of Bournemouth has been encouraging people to meet socially and use recreational technologies, such as the Nintendo Wii, DS and Apple's iPad, and reports very positive results (Innes and Cutler 2013). Similarly, a project in Sheffield explored the potential of iPads for leisure and recreation (Smith and Mountain 2012), with preliminary findings confirming the benefits that people can derive from engagement. Applications can go beyond gaming to the facilitation of hobbies and interests and enabling socialisation with others through features such as Skype and FaceTime. As with other interests and pastimes, personal interests and choice will determine the extent of engagement and the activities that are selected.

Who might this work with?

Case Study 6.1 – **Tom**,[1] with early to moderate stages of dementia

Tom received a diagnosis of dementia four years ago and is now in his late 70s. He lives with his wife Moira who is his main companion and also his carer. They have one son who lives nearby and a daughter who lives in New Zealand. A quiet, retiring man, Tom has become very passive and increasingly apathetic. However, he has retained his lifelong interest in jazz music, can be a keen talker and remains relatively independent, using several strategies (assisted by Moira) to combat his memory problems. Moira is highly sociable and can find the demands stemming from Tom's apathy combined with those resulting from his cognitive loss to be frustrating. She needs her own outlets for social activities but is reluctant to leave Tom; they previously did everything together and were keen members of a social history group. However, joint interests have now telescoped to going to an Alzheimer's café. They did have a volunteer to assist Tom with his own interests on a weekly basis for a short time, but according to Moira it was a 'disaster'. The volunteer was ill prepared and reliant upon Moira for suggestions of activities for Tom to pursue, which defeated the notion of any respite.

Tom would still benefit from some individualised structured activity each week that is independent from Moira and meets his specific interests. It may be appropriate for him to get involved in a work-based scheme for people with dementia if it is available. Alternatively, a volunteer could still provide one-to-one sessions as previously intended. However, a key requirement is taking time to get to know Tom, his past

---

1   Case study names in this chapter are pseudonyms.

and present interests and preferences and the local resources. One of the consequences of dementia is that abilities and motivation are highly variable, which means that the facilitator must always have a range of resources and options readily available to match the circumstances that exist at that moment.

Case Study 6.2 – **Eva**, with moderate to later stages of dementia

Eva, a widow of over 20 years, is 94 years old and lives on her own in the same house in which she raised her family. She has one daughter who visits once a week but who she is in contact with on a daily basis. Although Eva received a diagnosis of Alzheimer's disease three years ago, she had been coping with the effects of the condition for many years previously. Eva attends a local voluntary sector daycare centre and is collected three times a week by the service community transport bus. The centre provides people with moderate to later levels of dementia that live in the community with the opportunity to improve wellbeing, develop friendships and maintain existing skills. Eva considers the centre as her 'lifeline' as it promotes a sense of belonging with others who are experiencing life in similar ways.

Eva is an articulate woman who is an active spokesperson at workshops and seminars advocating for a societal increase in dementia awareness. This involvement extended to her participation in a research study exploring touch-screen computer technology in the promotion of enjoyable activities with people living with dementia. Eva was an enthusiastic and proactive participant who engaged consistently well in all of the new activities that were introduced during the research project. The supportive environment and opportunities to engage in enjoyable activities empowered Eva to achieve numerous goals, thus enhancing her sense of self-worth despite the stage of her condition.

Key features needed for implementation

- Increased awareness of the value of meaningful activity for health and wellbeing on the part of dementia practitioners.

- Access to a range of opportunities to maintain physical, mental and social wellbeing that meet the interests and abilities of the individual.

- Up-to-date, readily accessed information for people with dementia and their carers about such opportunities.

- Assistance to maintain existing social connectivity and identify and develop new contacts if possible.

- Identification of ways of promoting integration and social inclusion for as long as possible rather than focusing on segregated services and facilities.

- Realistic involvement of the family carer in shared social and recreational activities, but also identification of opportunities for separate pastimes.

- Activities and ways of participating that are not necessarily specialist and do not infantilise the person with dementia.

Recommendations for what works well and not so well

People with dementia value the opportunity to engage in activities that meet their personal preferences with the interests they might have, spanning the range of potential choices that exist within the overall population. Some activity adaptation may be necessary to meet the abilities of the individual, and the person may also seek to engage with new interests due to difficulties with undertaking what they previously enjoyed.

The emphasis in the early to moderate stages of the condition should be on normalising activities that can promote inclusivity rather than on therapeutic modalities that are usually more appropriate for those with advanced illness.

Activities that involve contribution and citizenship, thereby enabling the person to retain a sense of self-worth should be aimed for, but it is also necessary to consider needs for support and how they can be met. Existing evidence concerning novel initiatives designed to provide such opportunities suggest that they accrue relatively high costs for small numbers due to the supervision that may be necessary. How citizenship activities can be made more widely available to people with early to moderate dementia and delivered in ways that are cost-effective warrants further consideration, and examples of successful programmes, such as those from The Netherlands mentioned above, should be used to develop programmes elsewhere.

Enabling access to timely and appropriate information about relevant resources and potential areas for contribution and for socialisation is one of the keys to continued engagement with society. Identifying ways of conveying this information and ensuring that it is up to date should be a priority for memory services and others who encounter people at the point of diagnosis. Conversely, raising awareness about dementia within wider society should eventually lead to individuals being able more readily to access a greater range of resources and support.

People with dementia can have difficulties initiating leisure and recreational activities and may need carer or other support to achieve this. These demands may be acceptable to the carer or alternatively they may find such engagement to be highly demanding. Those involved in working with people with dementia and their carers have to be alert and sensitive to any prevailing challenges stemming from the relationship between the individual and their carer and adapt their approach in response. They also have to able to assist the carer with identifying strategies to sustain activity engagement in the person they are caring for.

The reliance that the individual might place upon their family carer for opportunities for socialisation can be high due to challenges arising from the condition and from the responses of society to dementia. Those without such support will be severely compromised and findings ways of enabling continued participation should be a priority for services.

It is only recently that the potential of technology for social and leisure activities for people with dementia has been recognised, with the prevailing focus still being upon equipment to promote safety and security. The ideal technology configuration for the future might be multipurpose devices that are able to respond to a range of needs, including leisure pastimes and interests.

Conclusion

Maintaining engagement in meaningful activity should be viewed as being an integral and important dimension of participation in dementia. While this chapter has focused upon the needs of people living in the community following diagnosis, this should not detract from the importance of activity for people at all stages of the dementia trajectory. The importance of involving individuals in activities of interest to them is emphasised, and there is a clear imperative to move beyond stereotypical interventions that are characteristic of an outdated model of dementia treatment and care.

References

Bartlett, R. and Connor, D. O. (2007) 'From personhood to citizenship: Broadening the lens for dementia practice and research.' *Journal of Aging Studies 21*, 2, 107–118.

Beard, R.L., Sakhtah, S., Imse, V. and Galvin, J.E. (2012) 'Negotiating the joint career: Couples adapting to Alzheimer's and aging in place.' *Journal of Aging Research 2012*, 797023.

Brodaty, H. and Arasaratnam, C. (2012) 'Meta-analysis of nonpharmacological interventions for neuropsychiatric symptoms of dementia.' *American Journal of Psychiatry 169*, 9, 946–953.

Bruin, S.R. De, Oosting, S.J., Kuin, Y., Hoefnagels, E.C.M. *et al.* (2009) 'Green care farms promote activity among elderly people with dementia.' *Journal of Housing for the Elderly 23*, 4, 368–389.

Clare, L., Rowlands, J.M. and Quin, R. (2008) 'Collective strength: The impact of developing a shared social identity in early-stage dementia.' *Dementia 7*, 1, 9–30.

Genoe, R. (2013) '"There is life after diagnosis": Dementia, leisure, and meaning-focused coping.' *Recreation and Society in Africa, Asia and Latin America 4*, 1, 1–19. Accessed on 20/08/18 at https://journal.lib.uoguelph.ca/index.php/rasaala/article/view/2716/2826

Hellström, I., Nolan, M., Nordenfelt, L. and Lundh, U. (2007) 'Ethical and methodological issues in interviewing persons with dementia.' *Nursing Ethics 14*, 5, 608–619.

Hewitt, P., Watts, C., Hussey, J., Power, K. and Williams, T. (2013) 'Does a structured gardening programme improve well-being in young-onset dementia? A preliminary study.' *British Journal of Occupational Therapy 76*, 8, 355–361.

Innes, A. and Cutler, C. (2013) *Evaluation of a "Technology Club" Programme.* Bournemouth Borough Council.

Kinney, J.M., Kart, C.S. and Reddecliff, L. (2011) '"That's me, the Goother": Evaluation of a program for individuals with early-onset dementia.' *Dementia 10*, 3, 361–377.

Kitwood, T. (1997) *Dementia Reconsidered: The Person Comes First.* Buckingham: Open University Press.

Menne, H.L. Johnson, J.D. Whitlatch, C.J. and Schwartz, S.M. (2012) 'Activity preferences of persons with dementia.' *Activities, Adaptation & Aging 36*, 3, 195–213.

Mountain, G.A. and Craig, C.L. (2012) 'What should be in a self-management programme for people with early dementia?' *Aging & Mental Health 16*, 5, 576–583.

Nygård, L. (2004) 'Responses of persons with dementia to challenges in daily activities: A synthesis of findings from empirical studies.' *American Journal of Occupational Therapy 58*, 4, 435–445.

Phinney, A. (2006) 'Family strategies for supporting involvement in meaningful activity by persons with dementia.' *Journal of Family Nursing 12*, 1, 80–101.

Potter, R., Ellard, D., Rees, K. and Thorogood, M. (2011) 'A systematic review of the effects of physical activity on physical functioning, quality of life and depression in older people with dementia.' *International Journal of Geriatric Psychiatry 26*, 10, 1000–1011.

Reid, D., Warnes, T. and Low, L. (2013) *Sheffield Dementia Information Pack.* Sheffield: School of Nursing and Midwifery and Sheffield Institute for Studies on Ageing.

Accessed on 22/8/2018 at www.sheffield.ac.uk/polopoly_fs/1.207026!/file/ SheffieldDementiaInformationPack.pdf

Robinson, L., Hutchings, D., Dickinson, H.O., Corner, L. *et al.* (2007) 'Effectiveness and acceptability of non-pharmacological interventions to reduce wandering in dementia : A systematic review.' *International Journal of Geriatric Psychiatry 22*, 1, 9–22.

Sabat, S.R. (2001) *The Experience of Alzheimer's Disease: Life Through a Tangled Veil.* Oxford: Blackwell.

Smith, S.K. and Mountain, G.A. (2012) 'New forms of information and communication technology (ICT) and the potential to facilitate social and leisure activity for people living with dementia.' *International Journal of Computers in Healthcare 1*, 4, 332–345.

Smits, C.H.M., Lange, J., Dröes, R., Meiland, F., Vernooij-Dassen, M. and Pot, A.M. (2007). 'Effects of combined intervention programmes for people with dementia living at home and their caregivers: A systematic review.' *International Journal of Geriatric Psychiatry 22*, 12, 1181–1193.

Sørensen, L.V., Waldorff, F.B. and Waldemar, G. (2008) 'Coping with mild Alzheimer's disease.' *Dementia 7*, 287–299.

Topo, P. (2008) 'Technology studies to meet the needs of people with dementia and their caregivers: A literature review.' *Journal of Applied Gerontology 28*, 1, 5–37.

Van't Leven, N., Prick, A-E. J.C., Groenewoud, J.G., Roelofs, P.D.D.M., de Lange, J. and Pot, A.M. (2013) 'Dyadic interventions for community-dwelling people with dementia and their family caregivers: A systematic review.' *International Psychogeriatrics 25*, 10, 1–23.

Wang, H-X., Xu, W. and Pei, J-J. (2012) 'Leisure activities, cognition and dementia.' *Biochimica et Biophysica Acta 1822*, 3, 482–491.

Whitlatch, C.J., Judge, K., Zarit, S.H. and Femia, E. (2006) Dyadic intervention for family caregivers and care receivers in early-stage dementia.' *The Gerontologist 46*, 5, 688–694.

Chapter 7

Goal-Oriented Cognitive Rehabilitation in Early-Stage Alzheimer's and Related Dementias

Aleksandra Kudlicka, Suzannah Evans and Linda Clare

Introduction

This chapter describes the rationale for applying a cognitive rehabilitation (CR) approach in dementia care and demonstrates how individualised, goal-oriented CR can benefit people with early-stage dementia and their families. The results of a pilot randomised controlled trial of CR in early-stage Alzheimer's disease will be discussed and case studies presented. The chapter concludes with a discussion on future directions for research and the possibilities for wider implementation of the approach into routine health and social care.

Cognitive rehabilitation and biopsychosocial model of disability

Cognitive rehabilitation is an intervention approach that focuses on enabling people with cognitive impairment such as dementia to achieve the best possible level of functioning and wellbeing. A rehabilitative approach is most commonly associated with physical, non-progressive conditions, but its principles apply to a much broader range of impairments conceptualised in terms of disability. The biopsychosocial framework for understanding disability (World Health Organization 1998) indicates that the impact of underlying impairment on everyday functioning (disability) is mediated by social and psychological factors. For example, environmental adaptation and social support may counterbalance restrictions brought on by physical or cognitive impairments. These secondary moderators may also exaggerate the impact of biological factors and lead to excess disability restricting social participation (handicap). The implication of the biopsychosocial framework is that a positive change may be possible even when the impairment itself cannot be removed, as is the case in dementia (Kitwood 1996). Improvements in everyday functioning and wellbeing can be achieved by introducing or improving strategies to cope with the psychological and functional consequences of the underlying impairment.

The cognitive rehabilitation approach derives from the biopsychosocial framework and offers a range of methods and techniques to bypass difficulties arising from cognitive impairment. Cognitive rehabilitation is different from *cognitive training*, which focuses on isolating cognitive abilities and processes by having the person practise a set of pen-and-pencil or computer-based tasks related to these abilities. The underlying assumption is that potential improvements resulting from practising the tasks will generalise into everyday functioning, with benefits for everyday life, but evidence generally does not support this assumption (Bahar-Fuchs, Clare and Woods 2013).

In contrast, cognitive rehabilitation focuses on practical solutions for well-defined day-to-day problems in the areas that are most relevant to the person with the impairment. It is highly individualised, practical and collaborative in nature, and it incorporates people's subjective perspectives on the illness and builds on their unique life experiences and coping strategies. An important aspect of rehabilitation is the identification of achievable and personally meaningful goals that would be relevant in the context of social functioning (Malec 1999). Working towards clearly stated, challenging but achievable goals directs attention and effort towards relevant activities, and enhances performance (Locke and Latham 2002). Goal-based approaches have been applied in numerous conditions, such as age-related frailty (Rockwood *et al.* 2003) and brain injury (Trombly *et al.* 2002), and have produced promising results in dementia care (Clare *et al.* 2010).

Cognitive rehabilitation in dementia

Considering dementia in terms of the biopsychosocial model of disability offers a helpful way to understand how various factors affect the presentation of dementia (Clare 2008). For example, personality and life experience will bring a range of emotions and coping styles that define the individual response to the diagnosis and the experience of cognitive decline. The experience of dementia affects not only the person with dementia but also people close to the person with dementia, and so the manifestation of the illness and the way in which people make sense of the cognitive change can only be fully understood within the social and family context (Kitwood 1996).

Considering dementia in terms of disability suggests that cognitive rehabilitation may be a useful conceptual framework for the design of interventions for people with dementia (Cohen and Eisdorfer 1986). Cognitive rehabilitation offers a broad range of techniques and methods that can be adapted to minimise the impact of memory and other cognitive deficits on everyday life. The potential for benefits from cognition-focused interventions is supported by evidence for cognitive and neural plasticity, which seems to be partially preserved in early-stage dementia. Cognitive rehabilitation may also build on cognitive functions that are relatively spared in early-stage dementia, such as implicit memory and semantic knowledge, and procedural memory for skills, routines and actions (Clare 2004). There is evidence to show that given the necessary support, people with early-stage dementia may learn and retain some new information (Backman 1992).

Development of goal-oriented cognitive rehabilitation for people in early-stage dementia: The pilot study

The feasibility of applying the cognitive rehabilitation approach in early-stage dementia was explored in a number of studies using single-case experimental designs or small-group pre/post comparisons (Bahar-Fuchs *et al.* 2013). Based on the results of a number of single-case studies, Clare and colleagues (2010) developed a pilot trial of individual, goal-oriented cognitive rehabilitation in early-stage dementia. The study employed a single-site, single-blind randomised controlled trial design with three study groups: cognitive rehabilitation (CR), relaxation therapy (RT), and treatment as usual (TAU). Cognitive rehabilitation involved eight weekly goal-oriented sessions conducted in the home setting. Relaxation therapy involved learning relaxation techniques over eight weekly sessions, which took comparable time and attention from the therapist for all participants. Treatment as usual included acetylcholinesterase-inhibiting medication, routine out-patient monitoring, and locally provided voluntary sector services, with all of these options available to the three groups.

Sixty-seven people with early-stage Alzheimer's disease who completed the initial assessment were randomised to one of the three study groups (CR: N = 23; RT: N = 24; TAU: N = 22). Forty-four participants were supported by a family supporter who also contributed to the study. Assessment included identification and rating of potential therapy goals and was repeated at three months and six months post-randomisation by a research assistant blinded to the participant's group allocation.

Goal performance and satisfaction ratings significantly improved in the CR group following the intervention, while there was no such change in the other two groups. The improvements relating to the identified goals brought some general benefits with regard to cognition, wellbeing and quality of life for people with dementia, and the wellbeing and quality of life of family supporters. Overall, the study suggested that cognitive rehabilitation may be an efficacious intervention to help people with early-stage dementia and their families to manage the impact of the condition. The key aspects of the intervention are described below.

Setting goals in cognitive rehabilitation

The process of identifying goals is an important aspect of the cognitive rehabilitation intervention. The first step is to identify areas of dissatisfaction by discussing the current situation and potential challenges related to particular aspects of functioning (e.g. everyday activities, personal relationships). The discussion clarifies changes that might be required and opens up common ground for the person with dementia and the therapist to collaboratively formulate specific goals. For the purpose of measuring change, current performance and satisfaction with the goal may be rated by the participant, the family supporter and/or the therapist at initial assessment, and then the ratings can be repeated at appropriate time-points. Before the therapy commences, agreement is reached as to what level of performance would constitute the full or partial achievement of the goal.

The goal-setting process requires a range of skills and experience in recognising and accommodating the individual coping styles of the person with dementia and responding to the dynamics within the patient–carer dyad. Discussing feelings may uncover areas of dissatisfaction and frustration, and elicit difficulties arising in day-to-day life, without the need for potentially intimidating problem-focused questions. It is usually helpful to talk about potential new activities, projects, and improvements that could be achieved, rather than focusing solely on problems.

The pilot study demonstrated that, with some help from a person familiar with the goal-setting approach, people with early-stage dementia can successfully identify practical and personally meaningful goals. Many people with early-stage dementia and their family supporters were prepared to talk openly about the problems they encountered in daily life, while others engaged in the goal-setting process with some hesitation.

Only two participants out of 69 visited by the researcher recognised their level of coping as optimal and did not set any goals. Reporting no difficulties in everyday functioning may indeed reflect relatively good adjustment to living with memory difficulties. It may also be related to limited awareness of memory difficulties and/or coping strategies (Clare, Whitaker and Nelis 2010). Given the collaborative nature of cognitive rehabilitation, the intervention has limited applicability where the person with dementia does not acknowledge any difficulties and has limited motivation to see improvements in everyday life.

The majority of goals set by participants in the pilot study focused on everyday memory functioning (e.g. remembering how family members are related) and on practical skills and activities (e.g. learning to use a mobile phone). Many goals were related to word finding and concentration difficulties (e.g. maintaining concentration, remembering names of familiar objects). A full list of goal categories and examples can be found in Clare et al. (2011).

Once the objectives of the therapy are set, the therapist can discuss with the participant possible strategies to achieve each goal, and collaborative discussion is used to ensure that the most feasible and personally appealing strategy is chosen.

Structure and delivery of CR in people with dementia

The cognitive rehabilitation intervention in the pilot study consisted of eight weekly one-hour-long sessions delivered in participants' own homes by an experienced occupational therapist. Between-session work on goals was encouraged and supported by the family supporter, where available and willing. The intervention was built around the goals set in the initial assessment, which were subsequently fully operationalised by the therapist, and included a number of strategies known to be useful in the process of rehabilitation in people with dementia (Clare 2008). Two commonly distinguished types of rehabilitative techniques are compensatory strategies and enhanced learning techniques.

Compensatory strategies

These are ways of getting around a difficulty in order to maintain a desired level of performance. As memory tends to be fallible, many people use some compensatory strategies, such as diaries, post-it notes and checklists, to remember important information. People with dementia may benefit from improving the efficiency of using such existing techniques, and from adopting some new solutions tailored to their individual needs. In addition to the traditional types of external memory aids (e.g. calendars, checklists, written instructions), there are numerous electronic aids to support independent living, such as mobile phones, electronic organisers and reminder systems. Improving the use of compensatory strategies and the implementation of new techniques may require extra training and practice, and can be facilitated by specific enhanced learning techniques (Clare 2008).

Enhanced learning techniques

These methods build on remaining episodic memory to re-learn forgotten information and make it easier to retrieve, or to facilitate better procedural memory functioning. People with early-stage dementia can learn or re-learn some new information, actions, skills and tasks to carry out daily activities. However, memory difficulties make this process particularly challenging for a person with dementia, and so enhanced learning techniques should be used only for important information and activities, and when compensatory methods are not appropriate. Enhanced learning techniques include a range of specific methods, such as action-based learning, or prompting and fading for various tasks and activities, and some simple visual mnemonic strategies, expanding rehearsal and semantic elaboration for learning and re-learning information (Clare 2008).

Other components of the cognitive rehabilitation intervention include strategies to improve attention and concentration, and to support better management of anxiety and stress. During the course of cognitive rehabilitation the therapist worked towards increasing engagement in daily activities and involving the family supporter. An important part of the rehabilitative process involved supporting progress and encouraging continued use of relevant coping strategies in order to maintain an optimal level of functioning.

Case studies

The application of cognitive rehabilitation is illustrated with two case studies from the pilot study. The first case study shows how it is possible to use enhanced learning techniques to improve performance on the individual's goal, and the second illustrates the use of compensatory strategies.[1]

Case Study 7.1 – Enhanced learning techniques: **Vera**

Vera was a 65-year-old woman with a diagnosis of Alzheimer's disease, with a MMSE score of 25 at the time of intervention. Her therapy goal was to learn to use a mobile phone to make and receive calls.

At the beginning of the intervention Vera was unable to use a mobile phone at all. She had been encouraged to use a mobile phone when going out alone, but was unable to retain and carry out the instructions given by family members. On a 1–10 scale (1 = unable to perform/not satisfied; 10 = fully able to perform/extremely satisfied) she gave the lowest rating of 1 for initial performance and for satisfaction.

To achieve the goal, one-step simple instructions were introduced (e.g. how to access the address book on her mobile phone). The therapist talked through the instructions whilst Vera carried them out. Recall was aided through repetitive practice of the task using expanding rehearsal. Once the task was mastered and recalled successfully after

---

1   Both case studies have been anonymised.

a minimum of 12 hours, the next step was introduced. The technique was modelled to Vera's husband to allow him to introduce new tasks between weekly therapist visits.

At the end of the intervention, Vera was able to make and receive calls, and receive and send text messages. She gave the highest performance and satisfaction ratings for her ability to use her mobile phone, and stated that she felt 'proud' of herself. Being able to use the mobile phone increased her social contact with younger family members, as she could exchange text messages with her nieces and nephews, and she was going out more often as her family felt more comfortable and confident about Vera going out by herself. Her family appreciated the technique used in the therapy and envisaged using it in the future to assist Vera with other novel tasks.

Case Study 7.2 – Compensatory strategies: **Sid**

Sid was an 81-year-old man with a diagnosis of Alzheimer's disease, with an MMSE score of 22 at the time of intervention. Sid was also the main carer, with support from social care services, for his wife Sara who had more advanced dementia. His therapy goal was to be able to return to continue tasks after being distracted. Sid described often being interrupted during daily tasks by the needs of his wife, and then found it difficult to return to what he was doing. In addition, he explained that he felt rushed and that he struggled with tasks that involved planning or needed more than one day to complete. He rated his initial performance as 5 and satisfaction as 3.

The intervention focused on the use of a whiteboard, with the intention that Sid could use it to make a note of what he was doing before tending to his wife's needs, and then refer back to it to re-orientate himself. In addition, a number of strategies were identified to address his attention and concentration difficulties. For example, tasks requiring his full attention were scheduled to be carried out when his wife was at a daycare centre, and at a pace that allowed him to complete them within one day.

Following the intervention, Sid rated his ability to return to a task after being distracted as 9, and his satisfaction as 10. His use of the whiteboard evolved during the intervention. He used it to record immediate tasks such as cooking times, and to plan tasks for the week ahead and record step-by-step achievements with these. He also spontaneously used it to help him get to grips with a new (and complicated) waste-recycling scheme introduced by the local council. He described feeling 'more in control' and 'less stressed'.

Outcomes and future directions

The promising findings of the pilot study led to the development of a large-scale pragmatic randomised controlled trial of cognitive rehabilitation, the Goal-oriented Cognitive Rehabilitation in Early-stage Alzheimer's and Related Dementias: Multi-centre Single-blind Randomised Controlled Trial (GREAT) (Clare et al. 2019).[2] The study was funded in the UK by the National Institute for Health Research (HTA reference 11/15/04) and aimed to produce definitive evidence about whether goal-oriented cognitive rehabilitation is a clinically effective and cost-effective intervention for people with early-stage Alzheimer's disease, vascular or mixed dementia, and their family supporters. The results demonstrated that cognitive rehabilitation is effective in supporting functional ability in the areas addressed in the therapy (Kudlicka *et al.* 2017).

The GREAT trial extended and improved the findings of the previous pilot study. An important implication of observing no difference between the two control groups (RT and TAU) in the pilot was that TAU provides an appropriate comparison condition for cognitive rehabilitation (CR). Consequently, in the GREAT study, participants (N = 475) were randomised into one of two groups, CR or TAU. Since performance on many goals continued to improve over the eight-week-long course of cognitive rehabilitation, it was felt that a slightly longer period of therapy would be more appropriate in order to fully establish and consolidate the benefits of cognitive rehabilitation. In the GREAT study, the cognitive rehabilitation intervention comprised ten weekly sessions over three months, and in order to maintain the benefits of the intervention, the therapy was followed by four maintenance sessions over six months.

The highly individual goals of cognitive rehabilitation require specific approaches to the evaluation of efficacy in group studies. In the pilot study, goals were elicited and rated using a structured interview, the Canadian Occupational Performance Measure (COPM: Law *et al.* 2005), which offers a standardised measure of performance

---

2   See www.exeter.ac.uk/great

across different individual goals. The goal-rating approach of COPM proved to be a sensitive and specific measure of change in the cognitive rehabilitation group, and the experience of setting goals with COPM in the pilot study informed development of a new comprehensive measure of change for goal-oriented interventions, the Bangor Goal Setting Interview (BGSI: Clare *et al.* 2012).[3] The BGSI is based on the principles of social cognitive theories of behaviour change (Bandura 2004) and incorporates influences from the concept of motivational interviewing (Rollnick *et al.* 2010). Goals are formulated according to SMART criteria: they must be specific (S), measurable (M), attainable (A), realistic (R) and time-delineated (T).

Inclusion of the family supporter, although not essential for successful cognitive rehabilitation, brings a number of benefits for evaluation of efficacy. Family supporters' active involvement seems to increase implementation of therapy principles between sessions, supporting the overall effectiveness of the intervention, and brings improvements in wellbeing and quality of life for the family supporters themselves. Family supporters' ratings add an informative dimension about the cognitive rehabilitation process, particularly where participants seem to overestimate their initial goal performance. In order to maximise information gathered in the GREAT study, all participants had a family supporter willing to participant in the trial.

An ultimate objective of the GREAT study was that if the intervention proves effective it should be promptly implemented into routine dementia care in the UK. Therefore, the final stage of the trial included development of a strategy to encourage incorporation of cognitive rehabilitation into NHS provision. In three research sites, the local services identified staff who could be involved in delivering cognitive rehabilitation interventions, and adjusted work practices to allow implementation of the intervention within existing services. The experience from the GREAT trial, and from the three pilot implementation areas, has led to development of the GREAT into Practice implementation (GREAT iP) project, funded in the UK by the Alzheimer's Society. In GREAT iP, the research team will work with a large number of NHS and social care organisations to begin the process of enabling services to offer this intervention to people living with dementia. A detailed strategy for wider implementation will be developed and this will serve as framework for implementing cognitive

---

3   See http://psychology.exeter.ac.uk/reach/publications

rehabilitation into other health and care provision for people with early-stage dementia.

In the pilot study, some participants became very actively engaged in the collaborative process of the intervention, and it is envisaged that some people with dementia and family supporters may be able to adopt the principles of cognitive rehabilitation intervention as a form of self-help following the course of formal therapy, or with just some initial support from a therapist. To support self-help efforts and supplement formal therapy, the team will develop information sheets and self-help materials for people with dementia and their families, with the expectation that these will be made widely available through the national Alzheimer's Society (England, Wales, Northern Ireland) organisation, which was a partner in the GREAT trial and funds the GREAT iP project. Finally, the team will work on effective international dissemination of the findings.

Conclusion

Goal-oriented cognitive rehabilitation is an effective approach to support a person's functional ability in relation to the specific goals addressed in the therapy, which may be helpful in reducing functional disability and maximising engagement and social participation. The approach has attracted the attention of memory services in the UK and internationally, and has the potential to be readily implemented by memory clinics. Most importantly, people with dementia themselves are interested in the development of rehabilitative strategies (Friedell 2002). The GREAT study provided much-needed evidence that cognitive rehabilitation is a clinically effective intervention for people with early-stage dementia and their family supporters, and initiated the implementation of cognitive rehabilitation into routine health and care practice. This may lead to a substantial improvement in the availability and quality of rehabilitative interventions for people with dementia.

References

Backman, L. (1992) 'Memory training and memory improvement in Alzheimer's disease: Rules and exceptions.' *Acta Neurologica Scandinavica, 85*(Suppl 139), 84–89.

Bahar-Fuchs, A., Clare, L. and Woods, B. (2013) 'Cognitive training and cognitive rehabilitation for mild to moderate Alzheimer's disease and vascular dementia.' *Cochrane Database of Systematic Reviews 6,* Art. No. CD003260.

Bandura, A. (2004) 'Health promotion by social cognitive means.' *Health Education and Behavior 31*, 2, 143–164.

Clare, L. (2004) 'Assessment and Intervention in Dementia of Alzheimer type.' In A.D. Baddeley, B.A. Wilson and M. Kopelman (eds) *The Essential Handbook of Memory Disorders for Clinicians* (pp.255–283). London: Wiley.

Clare, L. (2008) *Neuropsychological Rehabilitation and People with Dementia.* Hove: Psychology Press.

Clare, L., Kudlicka, A., Oyebode, J.R., Jones, R.W. *et al.* (2019) 'Individual goal-oriented cognitive rehabilitation to improve everyday functioning for people with early-stage dementia: A multicentre randomised controlled trial (the GREAT trial).' [Epub ahead of print.] *International Journal of Geriatric Psychiatry.* doi:10.1002/gps.5076

Clare, L., Evans, S., Parkinson, C., Woods, R.T. and Linden, D. (2011) 'Goal-setting in cognitive rehabilitation for people with early-stage Alzheimer's disease.' *Clinical Gerontologist 34*, 220–236.

Clare, L., Hindle, J.V., Jones, I.R., Thom, J.M. *et al.* (2012) 'The AgeWell study of behaviour change to promote health and well-being in later life: Study protocol for a randomized controlled trial.' *Trials 13*, 115.

Clare, L., Linden, D.E.J., Woods, R.T., Whitaker, C.J. *et al.* (2010) 'Goal-oriented cognitive rehabilitation for people with early-stage Alzheimer disease: A single-blind randomized controlled trial of clinical efficacy.' *American Journal of Geriatric Psychiatry 18*, 928–939.

Clare, L., Whitaker, C.J. and Nelis, S.M. (2010) 'Appraisal of memory functioning and memory performance in healthy ageing and early-stage Alzheimer's disease.' *Aging Neuropsychology and Cognition 17*, 4, 462–491.

Cohen, D. and Eisdorfer, C. (1986) *The Loss of Self: A Family Resource for the Care of Alzheimer's Disease and Related Disorders.* New York: W.W Norton & Co.

Friedell, M. (2002) 'Awareness: A personal memoir on the changing quality of life in Alzheimer's.' *Dementia 1*, 3, 359–366.

Kitwood, T. (1996) 'A Dialectical Framework for Dementia.' In R.T. Woods (ed.) *Handbook of the Clinical Psychology of Ageing* (pp.267–282). Chichester: John Wiley & Sons.

Kudlicka, A., Bayer, A., Jones, R., Kopelman, M. *et al.* (2017) 'Goal-oriented cognitive rehabilitation in early-stage dementia: Results from the GREAT trial.' *Innovation in Aging 1*(Suppl 1), 425–425.

Law, M., Baptiste, S., Carswell, A., McColl, M. A., Polatajko, H. and Pollock, N. (2005) *Canadian Occupational Performance Measure* (4th edn). Ottawa, ON: CAOT Publications ACE.

Locke, E.A. and Latham, G.P. (2002) 'Building a practically useful theory of goal setting and task motivation: A 35-year odyssey.' *American Psychologist 57*, 9, 705–717.

Malec, J.F. (1999) 'Goal attainment scaling in rehabilitation.' *Neuropsychological Rehabilitation 9*, 3–4, 253–275.

Rockwood, K., Howlett, S., Stadnyk, K., Carver, D., Powell, C. and Stolee, P. (2003) 'Responsiveness of goal attainment scaling in a randomized controlled trial of comprehensive geriatric assessment.' *Journal of Clinical Epidemiology 56*, 736–743.

Rollnick, S., Butler, C.C., Kinnersley, P., Gregory, J. and Mash, B. (2010) 'Motivational interviewing.' *British Medical Journal 340*, c1900.

Trombly, C.A., Radomski, M.V., Trexel, C. and Burnett-Smith, S.E. (2002) 'Occupational therapy and achievement of self-identified goals by adults with acquired brain injury: Phase II.' *American Journal of Occupational Therapy 56*, 489–498.

World Health Organization (1998) *International Classification of Impairments, Disabilities and Handicaps.* Geneva: World Health Organization.

Chapter 8

Managing Depression in People with Early Dementia

FINDINGS FROM A THERAPEUTIC TRIAL

Katja Werheid, Angelika Thöne-Otto, Johanne
Tonga and Alexander Kurz

Introduction

Feeling depressed is a frequent complaint among people with dementia. Using standardised diagnostic criteria, minor depression seems to affect about a quarter (26%) of people with Alzheimer's disease and major depression a further quarter (26%) (Starkstein *et al.* 2005). The prevalence of clinically significant depression is higher among people with mild and moderate dementia than among people with severe dementia (Lövheim *et al.* 2008). Depression is also common in dementia caused by cerebrovascular (heart) disease (vascular dementia) and fronto-temporal degeneration or Lewy body disease (Engelborghs *et al.* 2006).

The causes of depression in people with dementia are complex, presumably encompassing changes in neurotransmitters that are involved in the regulation of mood, as well as psychological responses to the loss of cognitive and functional abilities (Mintzer and O'Neill 2011). Irrespective of its origin, depression in people with dementia worsens cognitive and functional impairment, increases carer distress and promotes moves to long-term care settings (Zubenko *et al.* 2003). Therefore, treating depression is a priority because this may help improve the wellbeing, quality of life and functioning of people with dementia (Gaugler *et al.* 2009). However, antidepressants have been reported not to be superior to a placebo among people with dementia (Bains, Birks and Dening 2002; Banerjee *et al.* 2011). In view of the limited efficacy of pharmacological therapy and the potential for significant adverse events or side-effects, guidelines encourage psychosocial interventions for depression and other behavioural and psychological symptoms (Hort *et al.* 2010; NICE 2018). Over the past two decades two randomised controlled studies have suggested that behavioural intervention through increasing the frequency of pleasant events and positive interactions (Teri *et al.* 1997), and its combination with physical exercise and carer education about behavioural management (Teri *et al.* 2003) showed promise. A systematic review of six randomised controlled studies concluded that psychological treatments are effective in reducing symptoms of depression and anxiety in people with dementia (Orgeta *et al.* 2015). The use of external memory aids, such as memory books including a daily schedule and autobiographical and problem-solving information, has also been shown to enhance wellbeing by improving communication between people with dementia and their carers (Bourgeois 1993). The effectiveness of reminiscence therapy for reducing depression showed promise (Woods *et al.* 2008), although a large study of group reminiscence for people with dementia and their carers did not demonstrate efficacy (Woods *et al.* 2016).

This chapter outlines the CORDIAL programme as an example of a multimodal intervention programme combining psychosocial intervention strategies. The challenges of real-world implementation and adoption into practice are discussed.

The CORDIAL intervention

CORDIAL incorporates behavioural management, external memory aids and reminiscence. The intervention consists of 12 weekly one-hour sessions organised in six modules (see Table 8.1). All sessions are described in detail in a standardised manual, provided as a published book written in German (Werheid and Thöene-Otto 2010). The book also provides materials such as a memory aids inventory or an adapted list of pleasant activities, psycho-educative 'caregiver letters' (e.g. see Figure 8.1) and sections providing advice for therapists when encountering challenging cases. All materials can, by means of a password provided in the manual, be accessed online.

Table 8.1: Therapy modules M1-M6 of the CORDIAL programme

M1 Introduction, Goals and Preferences
M2 External Memory Aids
M3 Daily Routines
M4 Reminiscence Work
M5 Pleasant Activities
M6 Summary, Goal Evaluation

There are four thematic modules: M2 – introduction of a memory book as an external aid, M3 – implementing daily routines in order to ease feelings of memory overload, M4 – reminiscence work involving collection of autobiographical materials as a source of positive emotions, and M5 – implementation of pleasant activities. They are flanked by an introductory and a closing module, in which the person's individual goals and preferences and goal achievement are assessed, with a carer's assistance if needed. To help people with dementia get the most out of this intervention, they are given 'homework' at every session, provided in written form on working sheets. Homework for the first session of M2, exploring awareness of memory deficits and in preparation for the topic on memory aids is outlined in Figure 8.1. In addition, carers are invited to take part in half of the sessions, to support transfer into everyday life. In the introductory module, therapists are recommended to undertake an individualised behavioural analysis, in order to provide evidence as they develop the person's therapy goals. Thus, despite standardisation, the manual can be individually tailored to an individual's needs.

Worksheet 2: My Memory Aids

Here is a list of Memory Aids people tend to use in everyday life.
Please check/tick if you use it.

Memory Aids	Do I use it: yes or no?
Another person reminds me about things	Yes ☐ Who is it? _____ No ☐
Notepad, Sticky note	Yes ☐ No ☐
Pin board	Yes ☐ No ☐
Shopping list	Yes ☐ No ☐
Smartphone reminder	Yes ☐ No ☐
Calendar	Yes ☐ No ☐
(...)	

Figure 8.1: Example homework worksheet: Session 1 – M2 'Memory Aids'

The therapy programme was evaluated in the CORDIAL study, a single-blinded, randomised controlled clinical trial involving 201 people with dementia (Kurz *et al.* 2012).

What works for whom and in what context?

In order to facilitate implementation we consider next the people with dementia and the context of the intervention; the therapists who delivered the intervention; and family carer involvement.

People with dementia and setting

All who took part had a diagnosis of Alzheimer's disease of mild severity. They scored at least 21 on the Mini Mental State Examination (Folstein, Folstein and McHugh 1975) and were usually cared for by their family member or close friend. People who were taking symptom-relieving medication for dementia, antidepressants, and antipsychotics at stable doses could participate in the study. However if a person had an acute mental or physical disorder, such as depression, was undertaking ongoing psychotherapy or cognitive training, had a poor command of language, or was dependent on alcohol or substances, they were not enrolled in the study. In practice, the therapists using the manual reported that the programme might also be suitable for people with early dementia of other types, especially vascular dementia, Mild Cognitive Impairment not fulfilling the criteria for dementia diagnosis, and especially for people with mild to moderate depressive disorders, for people with sub-clinical depressive symptoms, or depressive symptoms that are part of the syndrome described as Behavioural and Psychological Symptoms of Dementia or challenging behaviour.

In the CORDIAL study, the setting for the delivery of the intervention differed: half the centres were at memory clinics and the other half were private neuropsychiatrists' practices. All centres specialised in out-patient diagnosis and treatment of people with dementia. The dementia diagnosis had been discussed with all participants and all were at least generally aware of their cognitive problems.

Therapists: Training and delivery of the intervention

The intervention programme was provided by trained behavioural therapists (psychologists or psychiatrists) with at least one year's experience in the treatment of older people and people with cognitive impairment such as dementia. They needed to have undertaken training in behavioural therapy, since the manual involves methods and techniques derived from behavioural therapy (e.g. behavioural analysis, modification of dysfunctional thoughts, and so on).

In contrast with manuals for treating psychiatric disorders, the CORDIAL programme was developed so that it could be adapted to a person's reduced cognitive capacities in the following ways:

- Sessions follow a fixed structure to support procedural learning.

- Instructions within the manual are short and easy to understand.

- Worksheets are clearly arranged, contain a minimum of text, and serve – because they are collected together in a file – as an external memory aid for homework.

Involvement of carers

In the CORDIAL programme, family or primary 'informal' (unpaid) carers have a central role, and it is difficult to consider how the programme would work without them. In each module, one session takes place with the therapist and the person with dementia, the other session also involving the carer, to help implement what has been learned or practised into everyday life. The carer, as designated by the person with dementia, is considered a co-therapist, who has a powerful role potentially in managing the challenges of everyday life with dementia, improving communication and strengthening social relationships. It is also important to enhance carers' care of themselves. To this end, in addition to attending 50 per cent of the sessions, carers receive written letters as an additional resource. These letters outline each module, provide examples of its implementation and include carer-centred topics. An example of a carer letter (Introductory Module M1):

Dear... [insert carer's name]

Welcome to CORDIAL! You and your relative have decided to participate in our therapy programme. I am looking forward to working with you both during the next weeks. Your participation is highly important, as you are the expert in the patient's everyday life, and you are also affected by his or her disease.

The CORDIAL programme consists of 6 modules with 2 sessions each, and needs carers' active involvement. You are welcome to attend every other session – that means the second session of each module. In the first session of each module, the person with dementia and the therapist start with a new topic at their own pace, and you will receive a letter. The letter contains an introduction to the new topic, some information, and food for thought around this topic that may be especially interesting to carers.

Tip: Find yourself a quiet moment and a comfortable place to read the carer letter. Perhaps a cup of tea in your favourite armchair? If any questions or comments arise during reading, please make a note of them and bring these with you to the next session, or reply to me. I will make sure that we will find some time to talk about it.

Alzheimer diagnosis – what next?

Receiving a diagnosis of Alzheimer disease raises worries and disquiet about the future. This is an absolutely understandable reaction, as many aspects of your family life will be affected by dementia. An Alzheimer diagnosis is not good news. However, sometimes it might bring some clarity. It may put a name on all the changes you have observed during the past months or years, and it might put an end to the uncertainty during the period of assessments.

(....)

Yours sincerely,

[insert therapist's typed first and family name and personal signature]

Implementation: Practical aspects

The CORDIAL programme is feasible in out-patient specialist settings in Germany (Kurz *et al.* 2012). A Norwegian adaptation has been tested in a memory clinic (Myhre *et al.* 2017; Tonga *et al.* 2016a, 2016b). However, it has not been tested in primary healthcare centres, daycare services or long-term care settings. In this section, we will focus on practical aspects when implementing the different thematic modules.

The reminiscence module is focused on positive memories, in order to support the person's sense of self-worth and to create a positive communicative atmosphere during reminiscence work with carers or significant others. However, if there have been personal tragedies, such as the loss of a child, abandonment by a beloved partner or exposure to catastrophic events, then working with biographical materials may reactivate grief and trigger depression. Another group, for whom reminiscence should be applied with caution, is younger people with dementia. People who have recently had to leave work, for example, may look back to what they were able to achieve only a few years ago, and this may reinforce their depression rather than their self-esteem. Therapists should be careful about these risks. Also, if someone has been married more than once, a new partner might find it difficult if the person with dementia focuses on the previous partner instead of the current relationship. In a case report, Tonga *et al.* (2016a) outline how a new partner felt neglected when 'Annie' (a person with dementia aged 59) talked about her first husband and their wedding. The therapist explained that it was important to accept all of Annie's experiences. Sometimes it may also be helpful to explain the temporal gradient of episodic memory to relatives, which leads to better recall of remote events compared to more recent ones. Therapists may point out that this does not mean that the person with dementia does not feel loved or would not prefer their current partnership.

Increased pleasant activities may sometimes be challenged by a person with dementia's apathy – this being a frequent symptom of dementia. In order to overcome difficulties in initiating activities, it proved more successful if these were embedded in some kind of daily or weekly routine or an external structure (e.g. a neighbour coming every Wednesday at 3 p.m. to take the person with dementia to a community café). As another example, the case of Mary (aged 77) who used to become very anxious when her husband was away from home, is described (Tonga *et al.* 2016 a). Here a weekly routine was established with the couple's neighbour, who came around once a week when Mary's husband went to the gym. Mary got involved in her hobby of painting during this time. This case is also an example of another challenge of the 'pleasant activities' model. In the CORDIAL manual, at least one weekly 'independent' activity is recommended, which is thought to be a useful step in view of the progression of the disease, when more paid or unpaid support is needed. Independent activities may be difficult especially for many couples who have been together for a long time. In these cases, it may be easier to reactivate or to continue positive activities – such as painting and going to the gym as in Mary's and her husband's case – rather than invent new ones. The reminiscence module may be another possibility for pleasant activities in cases such as Mary and her husband.

As a final practical aspect, the manual-based programme only lasted for 12 sessions across three months, due to the time constraints of the funding for the CORDIAL study. The therapists reported, however, that longer than three months was needed in order to achieve lasting behavioural changes. It is not always necessary to increase the number of sessions. Instead, the intervals between the sessions may, after an initial warming-up period, be extended. This may be especially useful when building up social and outdoor activities as part of the pleasant activities module.

Case Study 8.1 – **Christoph**[1]

Christoph, aged 69, wanted to join his cousin to go swimming in a group organised by a sports club. After an initial trial session, he had to apply for membership in the club and be accepted, and thereafter his carer daughter organised the journey to the swimming pool. These preparatory steps took three weeks. Only one session took place in this period. During this session, Christoph and his daughter were supported in problem solving. The subsequent session was scheduled after the first swimming expedition, in order to evaluate the new activity.

Evaluation and outcomes

The CORDIAL programme was developed as a multimodal cognitive rehabilitation programme not primarily aiming at improving

---

1   A pseudonym.

cognitive abilities, but at fostering coping with everyday tasks in the context of dementia. Accordingly, activities of daily living as measured by Bayer's Activities of Daily Living Scale (ADL: Hindmarch *et al.* 1998) served as a primary outcome measure, but the two groups (control and experimental) who were still living independently had high scores in this measure and did not differ significantly on this measure at post-intervention assessment, nor in six- and 12-month follow-ups. On the Geriatric Depression Scale (GDS: Yesavage *et al.* 1983), there was a significant antidepressant effect among women. Using regression analyses our statistical data showed that the antidepressive effect was pronounced among people with dementia with depressive symptoms as evidenced by a GDS score above 9 (Werheid *et al.* 2015), an effect that was later confirmed by the Norwegian Cordial study using the MADRS (Tonga *et al.* in press). We also found improvements in quality of life and treatment satisfaction among those who had participated in the intervention compared to those who had not. Additional assessments of self-efficacy (Schwarzer and Jerusalem 1995) at six- and 12-month follow-up showed a group difference. These could, however, not be controlled for baseline differences, as no baseline assessment of self-efficacy had been conducted. Other results of the study were that feasibility, treatment adherence and carer commitment were excellent, and drop-out-rates were extremely low, about 1 per cent.

Conclusions

The findings of the CORDIAL study may be helpful when designing further studies in several ways. Future research on this and on similar intervention programmes should employ more sensitive assessment instruments of everyday function. Assessment of personalised functional goals (Clare *et al.* 2010) might be better suited than the Bayer ADL scale. For self-report of depressive symptoms, the GDS and CES-D are recommended, and preliminary promising results on a self-efficacy scale should be further examined. It is conceivable that due to its psychotherapy underpinnings, the CORDIAL programme acts rather on participants' evaluation of the situation than on the situation itself, as indicated by the self-efficacy ratings. The most prominent effect of the CORDIAL programme was a reduction of depressive symptoms, which may also indirectly benefit cognitive functions. The CORDIAL programme might thus be especially well suited for people with dementia and depression. However, further research is needed on this point, focusing on people with depressive disorders in addition to dementia, and further exploring gender-specific effects (Baron *et al.* 2015).

Taking a broader view, evidence for a specifically antidepressive effect of multimodal interventions following a broad definition of cognitive rehabilitation is scarce (Bahar-Fuchs, Clare and Woods 2013), but there is initial evidence for improvement of quality of life and social relationships (Clare *et al.* 2010). Combinations of psychotherapy and cognitive rehabilitation approaches may be promising since most people with dementia and their relatives focus primarily on cognitive deficits, and consider depressive emotions as a consequence of dementia symptoms instead of potentially treatable. Thus cognitive rehabilitation strategies have the potential to increase people with dementia's and their carers' feeling of self-efficacy in dealing with the disease and reduce feelings of helplessness. Further research is needed here, especially on the effect of different types of intervention. In the CORDIAL study, participants took part in all therapy modules, so the antidepressive effects of this multimodal intervention cannot be attributed to a specific module.

References

Bahar-Fuchs, A., Clare, L. and Woods, B. (2013) 'Cognitive training and cognitive rehabilitation for mild to moderate Alzheimer's disease and vascular dementia.' *Cochrane Database of Systematic Reviews 6*, Art. no. CD003260.

Bains, J., Birks, J.S. and Dening, T.R. (2002) 'The efficacy of antidepressants in the treatment of depression in dementia.' *Cochrane Database Systematic Reviews*, Art no. CD003944.

Banerjee, S., Hellier, J., Dewey, M., Romeo, R. *et al.* (2011) 'Setraline or mirtazapine for depression in dementia (HTA-SADD): A randomised, multicentre, double-blind, placebo-controlled trial.' *Lancet 378*, 403–411.

Baron, S., Ulstein, I. and Werheid, K. (2015) 'Psychosocial interventions in Alzheimer's disease and amnestic mild cognitive impairment: Evidence for gender bias in clinical trials.' *Aging and Mental Health 19*, 4, 290–305.

Bourgeois, M.S. (1993) 'Effects of memory aids on the dyadic conversations of individuals with dementia.' *Journal of Applied Behavioural Analysis 26*, 1, 77–87.

Clare, L., Linden, D.E.J., Woods, R.T., Whitaker, C.J. *et al.* (2010) 'Goal-oriented cognitive rehabilitation for people with early-stage Alzheimer disease: A single-blind randomized controlled trial of clinical efficacy.' *American Journal of Geriatric Psychiatry 18*, 928–939.

Engelborghs, S., Maertens, K., Marien, P., Vloeberghs, E. *et al.* (2006) 'Behavioural and neuropsychological correlates of frontal lobe features in dementia.' *Psychological Medicine 36*, 8, 1173–1182.

Folstein, M.F., Folstein, S.E. and McHugh, P.R. (1975) 'Mini-mental state: A practical method for grading the cognitive state of patients for the clinician.' *Journal of Psychiatric Research 12*, 189–198.

Gaugler, J.E., Yu, F., Krichbaum, K. and Wyman, J.F. (2009) 'Predictors of nursing home admission for persons with dementia.' *Medical Care 47*, 2, 191–198.

Hindmarch, I., Lehfeld, H., de Jongh, P. and Erzigkeit, H. (1998) 'The Bayer Activities of Daily Living Scale (B-ADL).' *Dementia and Geriatric Cognitive Disorders 9*, Supplement 2, 20–26.

Hort, J., O'Brien, J.T., Gainotti, G., Pirttila, T. *et al.* (2010) 'EFNS guidelines for the diagnosis and management of Alzheimer's disease.' *European Journal of Neurology 17*, 10, 1236–1248.

Kurz, A.,Thöne-Otto, A., Cramer, B., Egert, S. *et al.* (2012) 'CORDIAL: Cognitive rehabilitation and cognitive-behavioral treatment for early dementia in Alzheimer disease: A multicenter, randomized, controlled trial.' *Alzheimer Disease and Associated Disorders 26*, 3, 246–253.

Lövheim, H., Sandman, P.O., Karlsson, S. and Gustafson, Y. (2008) 'Behavioral and psychological symptoms of dementia in relation to level of cognitive impairment.' *International Psychogeriatrics 20*, 4, 777–789.

Mintzer, J. and O'Neill, C. (2011) 'Depression in Alzheimer's disease: Consequence or contributing factor?' *Expert Reviews in Neurotherapy 11*, 11, 1501–1503.

Myhre, J., Tonga, J., Ulstein, I., Høye, S. and Kvaal, K (2017) 'The coping experiences of spouses of persons with dementia.' *Journal of Clinical Nursing.* doi:10.1111/jocn.14047

National Institute for Health and Care Excellence (NICE) (2018) *Dementia – Assessment, Management and Support for People Living with Dementia and Their Carers.* NICE Clinical Guideline NG97. Accessed on 3/8/2018 at www.nice.org.uk/guidance/ng97

Orgeta, V., Qazi, A., Spector, A. and Orrell, M. (2015) 'Psychological treatments for depression and anxiety in dementia and mild cognitive impairment: Systematic review and meta-analysis.' *British Journal of Psychiatry 207*, 4, 293–298.

Schwarzer, R. and Jerusalem, M. (1995) 'Generalized Self-Efficacy Scale.' In J. Weinman, S. Wright and M. Johnston (eds) *Measures in Health Psychology: A User's Portfolio. Causal and Control Beliefs* (pp.35–37). Windsor: NFER-Nelson.

Starkstein, S.E., Jorge, R., Mizrahi, R. and Robinson R.G. (2005) 'The construct of minor and major depression in Alzheimer's disease.' *American Journal of Psychiatry 162*, 11, 2086–2093.

Teri, L., Gibbons, L.E., McCurry, S.M., Logsdon, R.G. *et al.* (2003) 'Exercise plus behavioral management in patients with Alzheimer disease: A randomized controlled trial.' *Journal of the American Medical Association 290*, 15, 2015–2022.

Teri, L., Logsdon, R.G., Uomoto, J. and McCurry, S.M. (1997) 'Behavioral treatment of depression in dementia patients: A controlled clinical trial.' *Journals of Gerontology: Series B 52*, 4, 159–166.

Tonga, J.B., Karlsoeen, B.B., Arnevik, E.A., Werheid, K., Korsnes, M.S. and Ulstein, I.D. (2016a) 'Challenges with manual-based multimodal psychotherapy for people with Alzheimer's disease: A case study.' *American Journal of Alzheimer's Disease and Other Dementias 31*, 4, 311–317.

Tonga, J.B., Arnevik, E., Werheid, K. and Ulstein, I. (2016b) 'Manual-based cognitive behavioral and cognitive rehabilitation therapy for young-onset dementia: A case report.' *International Psychogeriatrics 28*, 3, 519–522.

Tonga, J.B., Bentz, J.S., Arnevik, E.A., Werheid K., Korsnes, M.S., Ulstein, I.D. (under review 2019) 'Managing depression in people with mild cognitive impairments and mild dementia with a multicomponent psychotherapy intervention: A randomized controlled trial.' *International Psychogeriatrics.*

Werheid, K., Koehncke, Y., Ziegler, M. and Kurz, A. (2015) 'Latent change score modeling as a method for analysing the antidepressant effect of a psychosocial intervention in Alzheimer's disease.' *Psychotherapy and Psychosomatics 84*, 3, 159–166.

Werheid, K. and Thöne-Otto, A.I.T. (2010) *Alzheimer Disease: A Neropsychological-Cognitive Behavioral Therapy Manual* (Original in German: Alzheimer-Krankheit: Ein neuropsychologisch-verhaltenstherapeutisches Manual). Weinheim, Beltz.

Woods, B., Spector, A., Jones, C., Orrell, M. and Davies, S. (2008) 'Reminiscence therapy for dementia.' *Cochrane Database of Systematic Reviews*, Art. no. CD001120.

Woods, R., Orrell, M., Moniz-Cook, E., Bruce, E. *et al.* (2016) 'REMCARE: pragmatic multi-centre randomised trial of reminiscence groups for people with dementia and their family carers: Effectiveness and economic analysis.' *PloS One 11*, 4, e0152843.

Yesavage, J.A., Brink, T. L., Rose, T. L., Lum, O. *et al.* (1983) 'Development and validation of a geriatric depression screening scale: A preliminary report.' *Journal of Psychiatric Research 17*, 1, 37–49.

Zubenko, G.S., Zubenko, W.N., McPherson, S. and Spoor, E. (2003) 'A collaborative study of the emergence and clinical features of the major depressive syndrome of Alzheimer's disease.' *American Journal of Psychiatry 160*, 5, 857–866.

Related reading

Aguirre, E., Stott, J., Charlesworth, G., Noone, D. *et al.* (2017) 'Mindfulness-Based Cognitive Therapy (MBCT) programme for depression in people with early stages of dementia: Study protocol for a randomised controlled feasibility study.' *Pilot and Feasibility Studies 3*, 28.

Spector, A., Charlesworth, G., King, M., Lattimer, M. *et al.* (2015) 'Cognitive-behavioural therapy for anxiety in dementia: Pilot randomised controlled trial.' *British Journal of Psychiatry 206*, 6, 509–516.

Chapter 9

Using Assistive Technology in Dementia Care

Franka Meiland, Henriëtte van der Roest and Rose-Marie Dröes

Introduction

We increasingly use technology to help with tasks and activities in daily life and work, to improve communication across distances and to promote safety. Dementia care also benefits from advances in the field of technology. Not only can it make care tasks easier or more pleasant to perform, but it can also help people with dementia to carry out some of the tasks and activities they would otherwise need other people to assist with or do for them. With the expected growth of the number of people with dementia and a simultaneous decline of resources such as staff, budgets for health and care, and accommodation and care in residential settings, assistive technologies may help bridge the anticipated care gap.

Assistive technologies can be defined as: 'any device or system that allows an individual to perform a task that they would otherwise be unable to do, or increases the ease and safety with which the task can be performed' (Cowan and Turner-Smith 1999, p.325). These technologies can be very simple, like a calendar clock, or more high-tech, like a sensor-based device working at a distance.

Technological advances for older people or people with dementia can be grouped together in different ways, four of which will be presented here. First, technological interventions may be classified according to application domains or categories (e.g. health and self-esteem; housing and living; mobility and transport; communication and governance; and work and leisure) (Van Bronswijk, Bouma and Fozard 2002). Second, they may be grouped according to their proposed impact or effect (e.g. prevention and engagement; compensation and assistance; care support and organisation; and enhancement and satisfaction) (Van Bronswijk *et al.* 2002). Third, they may be grouped according to the people who use the technology (e.g. people with dementia; family carers and professionals; or the environment in which technology is used: in the community or in long-term care facilities). Last, assistive technologies may be classified according to the needs of the target group they address, as the need for (personalised) information, the need for support with regard to dementia symptoms, the need for social contact, and the need for health monitoring and perceived safety (Lauriks *et al.* 2007).

Research among people with dementia living at home shows that their most frequently experienced unmet needs are located in the areas of information about the syndrome and care and welfare services that could assist them; other commonly unmet needs are support for memory problems, social contact, daily activities and safety (van der Roest *et al.* 2009). These unmet needs, except for memory problems, are also frequently experienced by older people with dementia in long-term care settings (Orrell *et al.* 2008).

This chapter critically reviews the current evidence for the range of technologies that could be implemented to help meet some of these most frequently experienced unmet needs. It offers a set of examples of the use of technology in practice and suggests that it has a rightful place in the range of psychosocial interventions that practitioners should consider.

Examples of assistive technologies
Information
Information on dementia-related topics to help family carers, volunteers and professionals in dementia care to improve their care skills is being provided increasingly by means of e-learning. A good example is the online course developed in the European STAR project.[1] This course is currently available in English, Dutch, Swedish, Italian and Romanian, and it is expected that it will be accessible in more languages in the near future. The course consists of eight modules, each addressing a specific topic in dementia care: the first two deal with dementia itself and with living with dementia, and are available at a basic level only; the other six consist of an intermediate and an advanced level where the topics discussed include dealing with the consequences of dementia, practical

---

1 https://courses.startraining.eu

support, and communication with people with dementia. The course has a mixed content: text material, videos, interactive exercises, expert interviews, knowledge tests and various forum groups (LinkedIn, Facebook). Research findings show that the STAR course is highly appreciated by family and practitioners since it is seen as easy to follow, the course material is well thought out, it helps people to carry out their care tasks more effectively and improves empathy and understanding (Hattink *et al.* 2015). An equivalent e-learning programme is the Open Dementia programme offered by the Social Care Institute of Excellence (SCIE) in the United Kingdom.[2]

New virtual-reality techniques enable family carers and professionals to experience what it is like to have dementia. These techniques were applied in the mobile simulator Into D'mentia,[3] which was developed in The Netherlands. Visitors enter the Into D'mentia cabin in the role of a person with dementia, and are guided through various everyday situations in which they experience the cognitive, emotional and social problems that people with dementia encounter in daily life. Another way to help people understand what it is like to have dementia is the 'Alzheimer Experience',[4] also developed in The Netherlands. This consists of a website which shows video clips of various situations that might be encountered in ordinary life by people with dementia. Each situation can be viewed from the perspective of a person with dementia, family carers or a doctor. One professional who works for many years in dementia care was surprised after her visit to the Into D'mentia mobile cabin. She now realised what it is like to have dementia. It changed her attitude. For instance she decided she would no longer talk about a person with dementia in their presence without including them.

The website Healthtalkonline[5] shows the personal stories and experiences of patients with various illnesses (including dementia) and carers. The information is based on qualitative research into health experiences, conducted at the University of Oxford. Various videos or audiotapes of interviews are presented, as well as reliable information about specific conditions, treatment choices and support.

---

2   www.scie.org.uk/publications/elearning/dementia
3   www.intodmentia.nl
4   www.alzheimerexperience.nl
5   www.healthtalkonline.org/Nerves_and_brain/Carers_of_people_with_dementia

Sharing information and support is one of the aims of the new developed Caregiverspro-MMD platform.[6] This platform provides both generalised and personalised information, alongside a social networking function. It is being tested from 2017 onwards in four European countries. (For more examples of informative websites that provide information about dementia and care and support services see the 'Useful websites' section at the end of this chapter – see also Lauriks *et al.* 2007.)

In two studies, positive effects were shown from the DEM-DISC,[7] a digital social chart of care and welfare services that provides information on services attuned to the needs of the user. In the group of family carers who used DEM-DISC both the people with dementia and the family carers had less unmet and more met needs (van der Roest *et al.* 2010; Van Mierlo *et al.* 2015). Also, the carers felt more competent compared to another group who searched for information without DEM-DISC.

Assistive technologies in the field of information about one's own medical condition, such as easy video consultation with doctors and other healthcare professionals (telehealth) are still very much in their infancy. In The Netherlands a pilot study was executed with a Digital Alzheimer Centre in which patients had access to their medical information and could consult neurologists at the Alzheimer centre of the VU University medical centre in Amsterdam. An evaluation study showed that the majority of the patients and carers were positive about the potential usability and usefulness of the online portal, but only a minority of patients found it easy to use (Hattink *et al.* 2016). Another example, not specifically related to dementia, is the Dutch MijnZorgnet,[8] a website that provides patients with a safe online environment to talk about their care, enables them to be in direct contact with their care providers, and to save and manage information about their care and health status.

Memory support

Many assistive technologies have been developed to support people with memory problems. These vary from reminders of the time and date, of past events, of appointments, and the time for taking medications.

---

6 http://caregiversprommd-project.eu
7 www.demdisc.nl
8 www.mijnzorgnet.nl

Examples include the Day Clock,[9] the Forget-Me-Not Clock,[10] and the COGKNOW Day Navigator.[11]

Also, people may receive video or voice prompts to help them perform daily tasks, such as washing their hands with the aid of the COACH system used in a care home (Mihailidis *et al.* 2008), or the steps in making a cup of coffee or tea (Lancioni *et al.* 2009). These reminder and support devices are considered useful as they improve orientation in time, provide structure for people with dementia and are reassuring for family carers.

Furthermore, there are various technological tools to train cognitive skills, such as Cognifit,[12] braintrainer applications and the Long Lasting Memory (LLM) training programme[13] with cognitive (Gradior) and physical (Fitforall) exercises (Franco *et al.* 2000). Preliminary study results of the LLM training programme show that participants find it useful and enjoy the sessions. A randomised control trial study in Spain showed positive effects on cognition from a multimedia cognitive stimulation programme together with day treatment and medication as compared to medication only (Tárraga *et al.* 2006). However, a recent review concluded that no significant beneficial effects from cognitive training in dementia could be demonstrated; better designed effect studies were recommended (Bahar-Fuchs, Clare and Woods 2013).

Social contacts and company

Support in maintaining or improving social contacts and company is provided by various tools for easy long distance contact with relatives or friends, such as picture-dialling phones, videophones and simplified mobile phones. Some are very easy to use for speaking and listening, with little action needed from the person with dementia. To promote social contacts, personalised multimedia bibliographies based on digital video technology may be used, such as DVDs with old films, music and photographs from the past that are familiar to the person with dementia and enable reminiscence activities (Damianakis *et al.* 2010).

---

9   www.day-clock.com
10 www.forgetmenot.no/english/forget-me-not-electronic-calendar.html
11 www.cogknow.eu/index.php/for-persons-with-dementia
12 www.cognifit.com
13 www.longlastingmemories.eu

Also, social robots like the seal Paro, the dog AIBO, and the dreamcat Venus may be used to enhance companionship for people with dementia. A recent review suggested positive effects of companion-type robots in the care for older people, including people with dementia, on (socio)psychological (mood, loneliness, social connections and communication) and physiological parameters (e.g. stress reduction), although the quality of the studies was judged to be poor (Bemelmans *et al.* 2012).

Engagement in daily activities

Digital music players, digital photo books or life-history books may support people to engage in daily activities. The prompts and reminder assistance for daily activities, as described above in the section on support for memory problems, can also assist people with dementia with their engagement in daily activities.

Furthermore, technologies such as the Nintendo Wii, Nintendo DS and the Apple iPad can be used to engage people with dementia and to promote social contacts, provide mental stimulation and encourage physical activities (Hicks, Culter and Innes 2013). A pilot study showed that people with dementia could learn to work with these devices and that they helped them to engage in enjoyable activities and promoted social interactions (Hicks *et al.* 2013). A recent review confirmed that people with dementia are able to use touch-screen technologies independently, but in practice 'more use could be made to deliver independent activities for meaningful occupation, entertainment, and fun' (Joddrell and Astell 2016, p.1).

Safety

With regard to support for safety, various global positioning system (GPS) personal tracking devices are available, as well as sensors in the living environments that can sound an alarm in dangerous or unsafe situations (falls, forgetting to switch off devices or gas, eclectic and water supplies, getting lost, and so on). Devices can be switched off automatically, or alarm messages forwarded to family or care organisations, which may follow up any call for assistance. These devices can provide independence for people with dementia and help them to stay in their own homes longer, and they may relieve family members.

Similar solutions can be installed in long-term care facilities with the purpose of enabling residents with dementia to move freely in various spaces (based on personal needs and possibilities) and reducing the time that members of staff have to spend on checking the people with dementia in their personal living spaces.

In the ENABLE project, various different assistive technologies were developed and evaluated, such as a locator for lost objects, a cooker alarm, an automatic night lamp to prevent falls, a night and day calendar and a multimedia music player (Cahill *et al.* 2007). Findings suggest that people with dementia and carers may benefit considerably from these devices In the ROSETTA project[14] the aim was to develop a multifunctional system for people with mild to more severe dementia living at home, to provide support for memory problems, social contact, daily activities and safety. The system consists of three sub-systems:

- the Elderly Day Navigator, a computer with a touch screen and mobile device for the person with dementia (with a calendar clock, reminders on the screen, picture dialling phone, digital photo book, outdoor navigation support and a help button)

- the Early Detection System using sensors in the home for early detection of behaviour changes

- an Advanced Surveillance System, with a movement sensor and camera for detection of falls.

The Elderly Day Navigator is intended for people in the earlier stages of dementia, and the other two sub-systems were designed to be used mainly by people in the moderate to more severe stages of dementia. An initial small-scale controlled explorative field study showed that people with dementia, family members and care workers considered the ROSETTA system a very useful development, and they made some suggestions of how to improve the user-friendliness of the current system, such as making it easier for family members to add appointments (Hattink *et al.* 2016). One daughter who used the digital agenda function in ROSETTA appreciated this function highly: in addition to including appointments, she also added little notes for her mother into the device. For instance, her mother used to forget to drink

14 www.aal-europe.eu/projects/rosetta

during the day. By adding a daily note in the digital agenda to take a glass of water, her mother appeared to function better.

Implementation

The likelihood of successful implementation improves if any assistive technology is accepted by the target group. For this to happen, it is important that the target group, such as people with dementia, family members and/or professionals, are involved in the development of the assistive technology (user-centred design). This promotes the development of assistive technologies that are attuned to the needs of future users. However, user involvement is not common in the field of assistive technology in dementia care (Span *et al.* 2013). From discussions at workshops with people with dementia, family members and dementia experts on the development of assistive technologies we have learned that it is important to take into account, for instance, specific dementia-related problems (regarding memory, orientation, understanding instructions, carrying out purposeful activities, recognising the meaning of pictures) and other physical impairments (such as vision and hearing problems, trembling) (Meiland *et al.* 2012).

The technologies must have simple to use interfaces that are intuitively usable, they need to be easy to configure for family members, and it must be possible to personalise them or to tune them to personal abilities, needs, wishes and preferences (such as adjusting the amount of information/ multimodal presentation/use of buttons or not functionalities). Another necessity is that the device should not be stigmatising for persons with dementia and not childish. Ethical considerations that should be taken into account in developing or using assistive technologies include an informed-consent procedure, addressing privacy issues, autonomy, changes in delivery of care and in the relationship between carer and care receiver, equal access to assistive technologies (rural and urban regions, differences in social economic status, home and long-term care, people living alone and with family members) (Niemeijer *et al.* 2012). It is also important that assistive technologies are guaranteed stable and safe before they are used in real-life settings (Topo 2009), that they are proven effective and that it is known for which target group the assistive technology is effective.

For implementation in health and care settings, it is also important that members of staff are properly trained in how to use assistive technologies in their work. Training of health and care professionals already needs to include attention to the value and limits of assistive technology in the field of dementia care, as well as ethical issues in its implementation.

Those supporting people with dementia need to be aware that some technological aids may only be used well by people with dementia if family carers are around to draw attention to this equipment or to help them use it. It would be even better if family carers themselves use the technological aids as well. Then older people with dementia may copy this behaviour, and as a consequence the use of the technological aids will not be stigmatising in their perception. One family in the ROSETTA project brought this into practice by using the digital picture-dialling function for all family members.

Outcomes

The examples mentioned above illustrate the broad range of assistive technologies that have been developed to support people with dementia living at home or in long-term care settings. So far, various positive effects of using assistive technologies have been reported in people with dementia and their carers. For people with dementia, these positive effects are more confidence, enhanced positive affect, increased communication and engagement in activities, enhanced feelings of safety and security, reductions in behavioural and psychological symptoms, increased independence, task engagement and safety (Bemelmans et al. 2012; Lauriks et al. 2007; Westphal, Dingjan and Attoe 2010). For family carers, positive effects have been reported on their feelings of burden, anxiety and depression, and improved competence and enhanced feelings of safety have been noted (Lauriks et al. 2007; Westphal et al. 2010).

However, sound research into the effectiveness of assistive technologies in dementia care is scarce, resulting in a limited evidence base. Examples of methodological limitations of current studies are small study samples, lack of (randomised) controlled design and shortage of long-term studies (Bemelmans et al. 2012; Lauriks et al. 2007; Peterson et al. 2012; Topo 2009; Westphal et al. 2010; van der Roest et al. 2017).

With regard to research on assistive technologies in dementia care, we need to improve the designs of effect studies, to focus on user-friendliness, usefulness, ethical issues and (cost-)effectiveness, and to allow for subgroup analyses to find out what technologies work well for which people in which settings. To promote research and collaboration on assistive technologies in Europe, the INTERDEM group on Early, Timely and Quality Psychosocial interventions in dementia care started its Task Force on Assistive Technologies in 2012.[15] This task force recently published a position paper on technologies to support community dwelling people with dementia (Meiland *et al.* 2017). In this paper, various challenges and potential actions were identified regarding development, usability, effectiveness and cost-effectiveness, deployment and ethics of technologies in dementia; many of which have been discussed in this chapter.

References

Bahar-Fuchs, A., Clare, L. and Woods, B. (2013) 'Cognitive training and cognitive rehabilitation for persons with mild to moderate dementia of the Alzheimer's or vascular type: A review.' *Alzheimer's Research and Therapy 5*, 4, 35.

Bemelmans, R., Gelderblom, G.J., Jonker, P. and de Witte, L. (2012) 'Socially assistive robots in elderly care: A systematic review into effects and effectiveness.' *Journal of the American Medical Doctors Association 13*, 2, 114–120.

Cahill, S., Begley, E., Faulkner, J.P. and Hagen, I. (2007) '"It gives me a sense of independence": Findings from Ireland on the use and usefulness of assistive technology for people with dementia.' *Technology and Disability 19*, 2–3, 133–142.

Cowan, D. and Turner-Smith, A. (1999) 'The Role of Assistive Technology in Alternative Models of Care for Older People.' In *The Royal Commission on Long Term Care with Respect to Old Age* (Research Volume 2 Appendix 4, pp.325–346), London: The Stationery Office.

Damianakis, T., Crete-Nishihata, M., Smith, K.L., Baecker, R.M. and Marziali, E. (2010) 'The psychosocial impacts of multimedia biographies on persons with cognitive impairments.' *The Gerontologist 50*, 1, 23–35.

Franco, M., Orihuela, T., Buenor, Y., Gomez, P., Gonzalez, D. and Woods, B. (2000) 'Computer for memory training.' *Journal of Dementia Care 8*, 14.

Hattink, B.J.J., Dröes, R.M., Sikkes, S., Oostra, E. *et al.* (2016) 'Evaluation of the Digital Alzheimer Center: Testing usability and usefulness of an online portal for patients with dementia and their carers.' *JMIR Research Protocols 5*, 3, e144.

Hattink, B.J.J., Meiland, F.J.M., Overmars-Marx, T., de Boer, M. *et al.* (2016) 'The electronic, personalizable Rosetta system for dementia care: Exploring the user-friendliness, usefulness and impact.' *Disability and Rehabilitation: Assistive Technology 11*, 1, 61–71.

Hattink, B.J.J., Meiland, F.J.M., van der Roest, H.G., Kevern, P. *et al.* (2015) 'Web-based STAR E-learning course increases empathy and understanding in dementia carers: Results from a Randomized Controlled Trial in the Netherlands and the UK.' *Journal of Medical Internet Research 17*, 10, e241

---

15 See www.interdem.org

Hicks, B., Cutler, C. and Innes, A. (2013) 'Using gaming technology to benefit people with dementia.' Alzheimer Europe conference, Malta.

Joddrell, P. and Astell, A.J. (2016) 'Studies involving people with dementia and touchscreen technology: A literature review.' *JMIR Rehabilitation and Assistive Technologies 3*, 2 e10.

Lancioni, G.E., Singh, N.N., O'Reilly, M.F., Sigafoos, J. *et al.* (2009) 'Persons with moderate Alzheimer's disease improve activities and mood via instruction technology.' *American Journal of Alzheimer's Disease and Other Dementias 24*, 246–257.

Lauriks, S., Reinersmann, A., Van der Roest, H.G., Meiland, F.J.M. *et al.* (2007) 'Review of ICT-based services for identified unmet needs in people with dementia.' *Ageing Research Reviews 6*, 223–246.

Meiland, F.J.M., de Boer M.E., van Hoof. J., van der Leeuw, J. *et al.* (2012) 'Functional Requirements for Assistive Technologies for People with Cognitive Impairments.' In R. Wichert, K. van Laerhoven and J. Gelissen (eds) *Constructing Ambient Intelligence: AmI 2011 Workshops CCIS. Vol 277.* (pp.146–151). Heidelberg: Springer Verlag.

Meiland, F.J.M., Innes, A., Mountain, G., Robinson, L. *et al.* (2017) 'Technologies to support community-dwelling persons with dementia: A position paper on issues regarding development, usability, effectiveness and cost-effectiveness, deployment, and ethics.' *JMIR Rehabilitation and Assistive Technologies 4*, 1 e1.

Mihailidis, A., Boger, J.N., Craig, T. and Hoey, J. (2008) 'The COACH prompting system to assist older adults with dementia through handwashing: An efficacy study.' *BMC Geriatrics 7*, 8, 28.

Niemeijer, A., Depla, M., Frederiks, B. and Hertogh, C. (2012) *Toezichthoudende Domotica, een Handreiking voor Zorginstellingen.* Amsterdam: VUMC.

Orrell, M., Hancock, G.A., Liyanage, K.C., Woods, B., Challis, D. and Hoe, J. (2008) 'The needs of people with dementia in care homes: The perspectives of users, staff and family caregivers.' *International Psychogeriatrics 20*, 5, 941–951.

Peterson, C.B., Prasad, N.R. and Prasad, R. (2012) 'Assessing assistive technology outcomes with dementia.' *Gerontechnology 11*, 2, 259.

Span, M., Hettinga, M., Vernooij-Dassen, M., Eefsting, J. and Smits, C. (2013) 'Involving people with dementia in the development of supportive IT applications: A systematic review.' *Aging Research Reviews 12*, 535–551.

Tárraga, L., Boada, M., Modinos, G., Espinosa, A. *et al.* (2006) 'A randomised pilot study to assess the efficacy of an interactive, multimedia tool of cognitive stimulation in Alzheimer's disease.' *Journal of Neurology, Neurosurgery & Psychiatry 77*, 1116–1121.

Topo, P. (2009) 'Technology studies to meet the needs of people with dementia and their caregivers: A literature review.' *Journal of Applied Gerontology 28*, 5–37.

van Bronswijk J.E.M.H., Bouma, H. and Fozard, J.L. (2002) 'Technology for quality of life: An enriched taxonomy.' *Gerontechnology 2*, 2,169–172.

van der Roest, H.G., Meiland, F.J.M., Comijs, H.C., Derksen, E. *et al.* (2009) 'What do community-dwelling people with dementia need? A survey of those who are known to care and welfare services.' *International Psychogeriatrics 21*, 949–965.

van der Roest, H.G., Meiland, F.J.M., Jonker, C. and Dröes, R.M. (2010) 'User evaluation of the DEMentia-specific Digital Interactive Social Chart (DEM/DISC).' *Aging and Mental Health 14*, 4, 461–470.

van der Roest, H.G., Wenborn, J., Pastink, C., Dröes, R.M. and Orrell, M. (2017) 'Assistive technology for memory support in dementia.' *Cochrane Database of Systematic Reviews*, Issue 6.

Van Mierlo, L.D., Meiland, F.J., Van de Ven, P.M., Van Hout, H.P. and Dröes, R.M. (2015) 'Evaluation of DEM-DISC, customized e-advice on health and social support services for informal carers and case managers of people with dementia: A cluster randomized trial.' *International Psychogeriatrics 27*, 8, 1365–1378.

Westphal, A., Dingjan, P. and Attoe, R. (2010) 'What can low and high technologies do for late-life mental disorders?' *Current Opinion in Psychiatry 23*, 6, 510–515.

Useful websites

www.alz.co.uk (carer information and information for people with dementia)

www.alz.org (Alzheimer's Association: information for people with dementia, and for carers)

www.alzforum.org (provides the latest scientific findings, maintains public databases of essential research data and produces discussion forums)

www.alzheimer-europe.org (Alzheimer Europe: tips for informal carers)

www.alzheimerexperience.nl (an interactive tool presenting the world from the eyes of a person with dementia)

www.alzheimers.org.uk (Alzheimer's Society: information about dementia, forum, various factsheets)

www.atdementia.org.uk (AT Dementia: information on assistive technology than can help people with dementia live independently for a longer period of time)

https://caregiversprommd-project.eu (information for people with dementia and carers, including details of final conference in 2018)

www.demdisc.nl (materials for carers and case managers)

www.forgetmenot.no/english/forget-me-not-electronic-calendar.html (electronic calendar)

www.interdem.org (pan-European network researching psychosocial interventions in dementia)

www.longlastingmemories.eu (Long Lasting Memories Project)

www.mijnzorgnet.nl (MijnZorgnet)

www.scie.org.uk/publications/elearning/dementia (Social Care Institute for Excellence dementia awareness e-learning course)

Chapter 10

Family Meetings to Prevent Mood Problems in Family Carers

Karlijn J. Joling and Hein P.J. van Hout

Introduction

Attending a programme of structured family meetings may help the 'primary' carer (i.e. the 'carer' most in touch with the person with dementia) to mobilise existing family networks in providing support. The assumption is that wider family support may help the primary carer to adapt to potential stress in caring for their relative. Within structured 'psycho-educative' family meetings, the positive contributions of different family members in support of the person with dementia can be maximised, thus preventing the primary carer from taking on the entire caring role. The mechanism through which family meetings might maintain carers' own mental health is explained by the stress-process and appraisal model. This has been used widely in research to describe the connection between stressors and health outcomes for family carers. By enhancing positive family aspects (ameliorating factor) and diminishing the negative aspects of family caregiving (secondary stressor) an intervention may improve the ability to withstand the difficulties of caregiving (appraisal) and reduce negative mental health outcomes (Joling 2012).

The effectiveness of family meetings was investigated by Mittelman and her colleagues in the United States (US) as part of a multicomponent intervention. In addition to four family counselling sessions, their intervention consisted of individual counselling sessions, support group participation and continued availability of ad hoc telephone counselling. This was effective in reducing carers' depressive symptoms (Mittelman *et al.* 1995, 2004, 2008), delaying relocation to nursing homes and having a positive effect on carers' quality of life (Mittelman *et al.* 1993, 1996, 2004, 2006). The intervention came to be known as the New York University Caregiver Intervention (NYUCI). It was combined with cholinesterase inhibitor therapy for the person with dementia simultaneously in three other countries, and showed positive effects on carer mood compared with those who received cholinesterase inhibitor therapy alone (Mittelman *et al.* 2008).

This chapter describes a 'family meetings' intervention (FAME – see Joling *et al.* 2008) that took place in The Netherlands (2007 and 2012), inspired by the NYUCI. The effectiveness and cost-effectiveness of FAME to prevent depression and anxiety was examined in a randomised controlled trial involving 192 family carers supporting a person with dementia (Joling *et al.* 2012a, 2012b, 2013). This chapter describes: the rationale for FAME; its application in The Netherlands; key features for carrying out the intervention; its outcomes, and what may or may not work. The chapter concludes with reflections for future practice and research.

The Dutch Family Meetings Study (FAME)

The effectiveness of using only the family counselling component to prevent mental ill health in carers was untested. Therefore, in The Netherlands, the family meetings (FAME) study investigated whether structured family meetings were more effective than usual care in preventing depression and anxiety in family carers. The effects on the severity of depressive and anxious symptoms, carer 'burden' and carer quality of life were also examined.

In the FAME study, carers began with one individual preparation session, followed by four structured family meetings that included their relatives and/or friends, and ended with one individual evaluation session. Ad hoc counselling was also available. Psycho-education was an essential component of the sessions, since early studies had demonstrated its consistent positive effects on outcomes such as carer burden, depression and subjective wellbeing (Sorenson, Pinquart and Duberstein 2002). The involvement of other family members in the intervention was thought to strengthen these positive effects. Thus the aims of the FAME intervention were to:

- educate families about the dementia including providing information carer support resources

- mobilise interaction with the existing family or social networks to facilitate emotional and practical support

- teach problem-solving strategies for coping with 'troubling' behaviour if this was present or if this arose in the future.

Implementation

We outline how to organise such a programme with families and highlight problems that may occur. Two anonymised case examples of families who participated in FAME are described in Table 10.1.

Table 10.1: Case examples

	CASE 1: Family A	CASE 2: Family B
Situation	Mrs A, aged 71, lives together with her husband who was diagnosed with mixed dementia about eight months ago. He had moderate dementia. They have five adult children who are all married. The family meetings took place at the As' family home or their daughter's home.	Mr B, aged 77, cares for his 78-year-old wife who has Alzheimer's disease (recently diagnosed at relatively mild stage). Mr B is most concerned about his wife's deteriorating functioning. He had to stop his voluntary work to care for her, which saddened him. The family meetings were organised in the memory clinic.
Participants	Carer, daughter, stepson, two stepdaughters, grandchild, friend attended (part of) the meetings.	Mr and Mrs B and their five adult children attended all meetings.
Family type (according to counsellor)	Mrs A has problems with the attitude of her children and experienced pressure. During the third meeting an old family conflict emerged.	Close family, socially involved. No conflicts about care or otherwise. The family has a relatively good understanding of dementia.

Content of the meetings	Main topics were how to cope with suspicion and apathy of Mr A. Learning to hand over care and to ask for help.	Main topics involved starting with day care for Mrs B, maintaining the couple's social contacts and asking for support from the children in case Mrs B has a 'bad day'. The children will do their best to be more aware of their parents' needs and to offer help.
Caregiver's evaluation	Mrs A had difficulties inviting her family. The sessions were burdensome and exhausting for her and arranging the sessions took too much of her energy. She decided to stop after three family meetings. She experienced no benefits. Her children always 'knew better' and did not want to see the deterioration in their father. Mrs A continues with support of her case manager who contacts her every two months.	Mr B had no difficulties in inviting his family. He experienced the meetings as useful. The children now have a better understanding about the condition and its consequences. They better spread their visits, which helps Mr B to manage the situation at home.
Psychological morbidity:	Scores at 0, 6 and 12 months follow-up	
Severity of depressive symptoms (CES-D score)[1]	19 – 21 – 24	6 – 9 – 9
Severity of anxious symptoms (HADS-A score)[2]	7 – 6 – 9	8 – 7 – 6
Burden experienced by the caregiver (0 = no burden at all, 100 = very heavy burden)	70 – 80 – 80	65 – 50 – 70

cont.

	CASE 1: Family A	CASE 2: Family B
Incident depression or anxiety disorder (MINI)[3]	Developed an anxiety disorder (agoraphobia) three months after baseline	Did not develop a depression or anxiety disorder up to 12 months follow-up

[1] The Center for Epidemiologic Studies Depression Scale (CES-D) ranges from 0 to 60. Scores of 16 and above indicate the presence of clinically significant depression.

[2] The Hospital Anxiety and Depression – Anxiety subscale (HADS-A) ranges from 0 to 21. A score of 8 or higher suggests the presence of clinically significant anxiety.

[3] The MINI International Neuropsychiatric Interview is a short, structured diagnostic interview for DSM-IV mental disorders, which was used to assess the incidence of depression and anxiety among carers.

Family meetings: Who attends?

Family meetings are organised to support a 'primary carer', meaning a carer who has adopted the main support of the person with dementia. Others who might be able to contribute to care of the person with dementia are also invited, including close or extended family, significant friends and neighbours. Although it is possible to organise a family meeting with just one relative apart from the primary carer, it helps to include more than one since this extends the range of support. During FAME, the counsellor met with, on average, four supporters in addition to the primary carer (range 2–14 people). This seemed to be a 'workable' number.

The counsellor and primary carer initially also discuss whether the person with dementia should attend the meetings. The FAME protocol did not include the person with dementia in the meetings, unless the family requested this or indicated that their relative was able to handle such a meeting. At the time we felt that involving the person with dementia might hamper open discussion of problems and concerns in families or cause difficulties for the person with dementia when problems that their relative had been encountering were discussed, or perhaps the person with dementia might feel overwhelmed in a large group meeting. If in doubt, the counsellor met the person with dementia as part of the meeting preparation to check out these issues. Other options included involving the person with dementia in the first family meeting and then deciding with them and their families, how best to proceed in subsequent sessions.

How to organise family meetings

Family meetings are facilitated by a counsellor who can offer psycho-education about dementia and has experience in running groups. FAME counsellors had postgraduate qualifications in nursing, social work, psychology or an allied profession, and were trained by the research team. One counsellor was assigned to each carer to build the relationship. Sessions were conducted according to a manual describing the family meetings in the NYUCI study (see Mittelman, Epstein and Pierzchala 2003) with our adaptation described in our counsellors' training and supervision protocol (see Joling 2012; Joling *et al.* 2008).

Preparation

Before the initial family meeting, the counsellor first meets with the primary carer to get an impression of the care situation, build mutual trust, prepare the carer for the family meetings, and introduce the notion of seeking help from family and friends. The topics addressed during this session include:

- explanation of the aims and possible benefits of the family meetings;

- definition and invitation of members of the carer's social network

- attendance of the person with dementia

- and the 'burden' of care.

The primary carer invites the people they want to the family meetings; for them, this can be an important step, as it could be the first time they are making others aware of the situation. If the carer finds it difficult to invite particular people, the counsellor can help by making the initial contact. It is important to talk this over with the carer (e.g. does the family member know the diagnosis?). Once the carer has decided whom to invite, the place and date of the meeting can be agreed. The family meeting can be held at a care organisation office or at the carer's home. Both options have advantages and disadvantages. Overall it needs to be as easy as possible for people to attend the meetings.

Family meetings

Often, a month or two passes before the family meeting is organised. During the first family meeting their purpose, the protocol, ground rules and the counsellor's role are explained to those attending. Everyone is invited to give their view on the situation and raise questions or issues (e.g. management of behavioural problems, uncertainty about the course and the prognosis of dementia, finding good-quality services, coping with feelings of guilt, communication between family members), since not all in the care system experience the same problems or have the same needs. Therefore, the meeting's content is guided by the primary carer's needs.

Although no standard themes are defined, the counsellor works flexibly with the general agenda described in the manual to structure the meetings (see 'Related reading' for the manual, in Dutch). The counsellor guides the family to devise ideas to help the carer and to delegate tasks. Follow-up meetings review the previous session, previous commitments and progress. During these sessions, some issues may be resolved, others become a priority or new problems and conflicts may emerge. These are then discussed in the same way as in the first session. Following the final family session, the counsellor and primary carer meet to evaluate satisfaction and to consider additional support.

Number of family meetings and timing

It is not clear how many sessions should be offered, or when is the best time to start. This depends on the family's needs. In the FAME study, meetings were held once every two to three months for 12 months. Mittelman and colleagues (2008) found that three family meetings could have positive effects. In FAME we noted that sometimes just one family meeting can trigger other family members to make substantial efforts to support their relative.

Barriers to participation

Initially, the carer can experience difficulty in engaging with family meetings. In FAME, many carers refused to participate in the programme. Most were due to carers' claims that the intervention was unnecessary since they used other services, or could (still) manage on their own, or did not see the benefits of the intervention. Many carers thought it would be too burdensome to add meetings to their daily tasks. Our additional impression was that refusal was often related to carers' desire not to burden their family or their relative with dementia, particularly when this person was suspicious of 'interference'. Only a few carers indicated any difficulty in talking to others about their relatives' dementia. A good explanation about the purpose and possible benefits of family meetings at the start may have overturned reluctance, particularly if this included different options on involving the person with dementia if necessary, or flexible arrangements for other family members to join.

Topics and reported benefits

Topics that are often addressed include: coping with behavioural changes in the person with dementia, changing relationship between the carer and the person with dementia, the burden of daily care, uncertainty about the future, how to accept support, how to express needs, and whether to start day care or long-term care moves. Despite some initial trepidation, most carers were positive about the intervention once they had been engaged in meetings. Benefits that were mentioned included: taking time with the family to talk about the situation without having the person with dementia around; better insight for the family about what dementia involves; more openness and listening more to each other; and having time to deal consciously with the situation, with professional help on hand.

Translation to other contexts

The structure of the intervention permits flexibility of content, making it an ideal intervention for diverse cultures. Nevertheless, translating an intervention to another country poses challenges. The standard care in The Netherlands is good and many supportive services are available. In the FAME study, participants in the 'usual care' group were free to seek out support on their own. Although usual care in The Netherlands may consist of different healthcare and welfare services, family meetings are rarely organised and seldom structured, with follow-up sessions. If organised, they tend to focus on providing clinical information and not on increasing family support and directly addressing carer needs.

Prior to this study, our pilot study explored how family meetings could be delivered in the Dutch context, and we adapted some of the NYUCI study protocols. For example, the NYUCI study was conducted only with spouse carers who were supporting people with Alzheimer-type dementia. It measured effects on depression but not on anxiety. In our study we included other family members (e.g. adult child, brother or sister), but the primary carer had to live together with the person with dementia or provide substantial care. We expected that these carers (and in particular children) could also be vulnerable to developing depression or an anxiety disorder. We also included people with non-Alzheimer-type dementias, since all dementia carers can have similar needs, such as coping with behavioural problems. The original NYUCI timeframe – six counselling sessions within four months after intake – was extended to about 12 months due to findings from our pilot that carers and family members preferred more time between sessions. Therefore, we chose a longer time span of two to three months between sessions. Evaluation forms indicated that most carers were satisfied with the number and frequency of the sessions.

The flexible structure of the family meetings intervention allows implementation in diverse environments. We worked in diverse settings: memory clinics, services delivering case management, general practices, home care settings and meetings centres for people with dementia and their carers. The clinical skills of the counsellors were rather similar. If a counsellor felt uncertain, they were assisted by an experienced counsellor during the first meeting. It seemed to help carer participation if the counsellor was already familiar to them. A prerequisite was that the family was aware of the dementia diagnosis. This made it possible to better target information and psycho-education and made it easier to talk about the course of dementia.

Our learning from the FAME study suggests five key strategies for use in family meetings:

1. Start the planning of a meeting early. It often takes time for the carer to get the family together. Try to plan a subsequent meeting immediately at the end of a meeting.

2. Prepare the first family meeting with the carer carefully. Explain its purpose and tell the carer what to expect. Carers often start without specific expectations. Prior to the meetings, discuss with the carer what they want to achieve from them. You can get back to this during the family meetings and help the carer to formulate their demands if needed.

3. Try to organise at least one family meeting without the person with dementia. Carers and family members often find it difficult to talk about problems when the person in question is around.

4. Try to be as flexible as possible (regarding time and place). This increases the likelihood of organising the sessions successfully, especially if family members are still working.

5. Try to stimulate the family to discuss issues and find solutions, but do not take a leading role in this. Do not be afraid of silences during the meetings.

Outcomes of the FAME study

The effectiveness and cost-effectiveness of the family meetings intervention have been described in detail (Joling *et al.* 2012a, 2012b, 2013). There were substantial levels of depression and anxiety in this sample of carers where almost 40 per cent developed this within 12 months. The intervention did not prevent the onset of depression or anxiety disorders; or reduce symptom levels and caregiver burden; or postpone the move of people with dementia to long-term care compared with those receiving usual care; or appear cost-effective compared with usual care in The Netherlands. We discovered that high numbers of family carers declined our offer to join the study, since they did not perceive the need for this intervention. Most carers who started the intervention programme were satisfied and experienced the family meetings as useful. About half of the carers in the intervention group completed the programme according to the protocol. Comparison of these 'adherers' with the usual care group revealed no other effects. No subgroups of carers who had a particular positive or negative response to the intervention were identified.

Implementing effective interventions

The NYUCI intervention (Mittelman *et al.* 1995, 2004, 2008) showed statistically significant but not very large effects on depressive symptoms in caregivers and had considerably delayed admissions to nursing home (Mittelman *et al.* 1993; 1996; 2004; 2006). This begs the question: Why did our family meetings intervention study not establish any statistical significant or clinically relevant effects? Next we will consider key ingredients learned from FAME that should be taken into account when implementing interventions in other contexts.

- *Consider the degree of contrast with usual care.* 'Usual care' participants FAME were free to seek out support on their own. Standard care in The Netherlands is quite extensive and many supportive services are available to carers. Over half (57%) of carers in both the intervention and usual care group in our study were already receiving additional counselling from a case manager. The higher level of standard care in some regions of The Netherlands may have contributed to limited contrast between the intervention and 'usual care', since benefits of the family meetings were not large enough compared with those gained from usual care.

- *Consider delivery of the intervention and its potential uptake.* Unlike the controlled setting of the NYUCI study with its own group of counsellors, we worked in diverse settings to implement the intervention into the daily practice of variety of counsellors. Potential reduced adherence by counsellors might explain the described lack of effect, but our analyses did not suggest that better adherence would have altered this.

  We ensured that carers entering the study were willing to take part, but the number that actually participated in the full intervention was relatively low and some carers who joined the study had no family meetings at all. Thus actually engaging in an intervention may not be the same as initial willingness. It would be interesting to investigate this finding in more detail to inform the development of future interventions.

- *Consider the intensity and dosage of the intervention.* Interventions that provide more treatment generally have better outcomes (Zarit *et al.* 1998). In carer research, even single-component interventions tend to have stronger effects than less intensive multicomponent interventions if they last longer or involve more frequent interactions (Brodaty, Green and Koschera 2003; Pinquart and Sorensen 2006). Some families only completed the intervention shortly before the last measurement and some were still participating in the intervention programme. This might have undermined the true effects of the intervention where data was collected at 12 months. A higher intensity may have led to more positive outcomes. On the other hand, counsellors in the family meetings study reported that it was sometimes hard to plan the family sessions, particularly when carers and/or family members had a job or lived in another region; and many did not complete the maximum number of sessions, although most were satisfied with them. Taking this into consideration, it is doubtful whether a more intensive intervention would have been feasible or necessary.

- *Consider the target sample.* This intervention was designed to prevent development of mood disorders in dementia carers who have a known vulnerability compared with those caring for a relative without dementia (Joling *et al.* 2010). All carers free from a mental disorder at intake, regardless of their level of symptoms were included. Additional analyses of carers with clinically relevant depressive or anxiety symptoms at baseline did not indicate added benefit from this particular intervention. However, matching intervention intensities and dosages to important risk indicators, such as levels of carer symptoms (Joling *et al.* 2012c) or levels of behavioural symptoms in the relative, is perhaps a more relevant way of supporting carers. For example, a study in the US only enrolled carers who had at least moderate levels of strain in their role (Belle *et al.* 2006). Outcomes were more positive compared to an earlier study from the same research group.

- *Consider alternative outcome measures.* We did not achieve measurable effectiveness on outcomes measured, but we did not measure the effects of other potential important outcomes such as feeling trapped in their situation, guilt and family relationships.

Conclusions

In contrast to the NYUCI study, the FAME study did not show statistically or clinically significant measurable effects of family meetings compared with usual care. FAME was methodologically strong with: a relatively large sample size; good blinded random allocation procedures; blinded interviewer data collection; and little loss to follow-up, mostly due to poor physical health in the carer. The FAME study has demonstrated that in practice delivering intensive family meetings over a short time period for all carers to prevent future mood problems is probably not feasible in The Netherlands. The feasibility of intensive family meetings alone, delivered over a shorter period for subgroups of carers with particular therapeutic needs could be studied further.

The context of the intervention was different to NYUCI: FAME counsellors were drawn from a variety of settings; FAME went beyond the spouse or a primary carer to engage with the broader family or significant social network; and 'usual care' in FAME may have been of a high standard of carer support.

Many carers felt they were supported by, and satisfied with, this intervention, but others appeared to have difficulty in finding time and other resources within their lives, to actively participate in meetings. This demonstrates the diversity of modern life in family caregiving populations, where different types and intensity of support, including family meetings may be needed. Our data did not allow us to examine in depth who this intervention might work for and when, as we did not have information on the range of personal aspects (such as carer coping styles) to inform us on who might benefit more from family meetings than others. The finding that carers with limited family support prior to the intervention were more satisfied with family meetings suggests that family meetings better meet the needs of carers when they feel they lack family support.

Future research on the value of family meetings in dementia could study: what the nature of 'usual care' in a given locality might be in terms of carer support; the timing of when a family meeting is organised and for what purpose (e.g. the time of diagnosis might be a time to engage families in thinking about future support of the primary carer – see Chapter 2); the effects of organising family meetings for specific subgroups of carers with a particular therapeutic purpose; whether the intervention effectiveness may be derived from its multicomponent nature including from tailored combinations of individual and family meeting support; and, following family meetings, whether longer-term availability of the counsellor who knows the situation has benefits for particular care subgroups.

References

Belle, S.H., Burgio, L., Burns, R.., Coon, D. *et al.* (2006) 'Enhancing the quality of life of dementia caregivers from different ethnic or racial groups: A randomized, controlled trial.' *Annals of Internal Medicine 145*, 10, 727–738.

Brodaty. H., Green, A. and Koschera, A. (2003) 'Meta-analysis of psychosocial interventions for caregivers of people with dementia.' *Journal of the American Geriatrics Society 51*, 5, 657–664.

Joling, K.J., van Hout, H.P., Scheltens, P., Vernooij-Dassen, M. *et al.*(2008) '(Cost)-effectiveness of family meetings on indicated prevention of anxiety and depressive symptoms and disorders of primary family caregivers of patients with dementia: Design of a randomized controlled trial.' *BMC Geriatrics 8*, 2.

Joling, K.J., Van Hout, H.P., Schellevis, F.G., van der Horst, H.E. *et al.* (2010) 'Incidence of depression and anxiety in the spouses of patients with dementia: A naturalistic cohort study of recorded morbidity with a 6-year follow-up.' *American Journal of Geriatric Psychiatry 18*, 2, 146–153.

Joling, K.J. (2012) *Depression and Anxiety in Family Caregivers of Persons with Dementia.* PhD thesis. Amsterdam: VU University Medical Center; EMGO Institute for Health and Care Research.

Joling, K.J., van Marwijk, H.W., Smit, F., van der Horst, H.E. *et al.* (2012a) 'Does a family meetings intervention prevent depression and anxiety in family caregivers of dementia patients? A randomized trial.' *PLoS One, 7*, 1, e30936.

Joling, K.J., van Marwijk, H.W., van der Horst, H.E., Scheltens, P. *et al.* (2012b) 'Effectiveness of family meetings for family caregivers on delaying time to nursing home placement of dementia patients: A randomized trial.' *PLoS One 7*, 8, e42145.

Joling, K.J., Smit, F., van Marwijk, H.W.J., van der Horst, H.E. *et al.* (2012c) 'Identifying target groups for the prevention of depression among caregivers of dementia patients.' *International Psychogeriatrics 24*, 2, 298–306.

Joling, K.J., Bosmans, J.E., van Marwijk, H.W., van der Horst, H.E. *et al.* (2013) 'The cost-effectiveness of a family meetings intervention to prevent depression and anxiety in family caregivers of patients with dementia: A randomized trial.' *Trials 14*, 305.

Mittelman, MS., Ferris, SH., Steinberg, G., Shulman, E. *et al.* (1993) 'An intervention that delays institutionalization of Alzheimer's disease patients: Treatment of spouse-caregivers.' *The Gerontologist 33*, 6, 730–740.

Mittelman, M.S., Ferris, S.H., Shulman, E., Steinberg, G. *et al.* (1995) 'A comprehensive support program: Effect on depression in spouse-caregivers of AD patients.' *The Gerontologist 35*, 6, 792–802.

Mittelman, M.S., Ferris, S.H., Shulman, E., Steinberg, G. and Levin, B. (1996) 'A family intervention to delay nursing home placement of patients with Alzheimer disease: A randomized controlled trial.' *Journal of the American Geriatric Association 276*, 21, 1725–1731.

Mittelman, M.S., Epstein, C. and Pierzchala, A. (2003) *Counseling the Alzheimer's Caregiver: A Resource for Health Care Professionals.* Chicago: AMA Press.

Mittelman, M.S., Roth, D.L., Coon, D.W. and Haley, W.E. (2004) 'Sustained benefit of supportive intervention for depressive symptoms in caregivers of patients with Alzheimer's disease.' *American Journal of Psychiatry 161*, 5, 850–856.

Mittelman, M.S., Haley, W.E., Clay, O.J. and Roth, D.L. (2006) 'Improving caregiver well-being delays nursing home placement of patients with Alzheimer disease.' *Neurology 67*, 9, 1592–1599.

Mittelman, M.S., Brodaty, H., Wallen, A.S. and Burns, A. (2008) 'A three-country randomized controlled trial of a psychosocial intervention for caregivers combined with pharmacological treatment for patients with Alzheimer disease: Effects on caregiver depression.' *American Journal of Geriatric Psychiatry 16*, 11, 893–904.

Pinquart, M. and Sorensen, S. (2006) 'Helping caregivers of persons with dementia: Which interventions work and how large are their effects?' *International Psychogeriatrics 18*, 4, 577–595.

Sorensen, S., Pinquart, M. and Duberstein, P. (2002) 'How effective are interventions with caregivers? An updated meta-analysis.' *The Gerontologist 42*, 3, 356–372.

Zarit, S.H., Stephens, M.A., Townsend, A. and Greene, R. (1998) 'Stress reduction for family caregivers: Effects of adult day care use.' *Journals of Gerontology: Series B 53*, 5, S267–S277.

Related reading (in Dutch)

Joling K.J. *et al.* (2007) *Handleiding Familiegesprekken.* [Family meetings manual.] VU Medical Center Amsterdam. Accessed on 13/08/2018 at www.vumc.nl/afdelingen-the mas/49661/27797/7341279/154786/Handleiding_Familiegesprekk1.pdf

Joling, K.J. and van Hout H.P.J. (2009) 'Ondersteuning voor mantelzorgers van dementerenden: Het belang van familiegesprekken.' [Support for caregivers of persons with dementia: The value of family meetings.] *Bijblijven 25*, 8.

PART 2

Reducing Disability: Care System Support

This part of the book covers evidence-based support programmes, when the 'journey gets tough'. The chapters outline support for people living at home as well as for people living in nursing or care homes. The interventions focus on support and skills of care practitioners and families to help with unmet psychosocial need and thus maintain health and wellbeing. These chapters are relevant when the person living with dementia has difficulty in communicating in an easily understood way, and when families and staff may therefore benefit from specialist programmes to assist them in delivering care and helping with communication.

Chapter 11

Supporting the Supporters

INTERVENTIONS TO REDUCE FAMILY DISTRESS

Ingun Ulstein, Jill Manthorpe and Esme Moniz-Cook

Introduction

Distress associated with the challenges of symptoms associated with dementia has various meanings in practice. In Scotland the term 'stress' and 'distress' has been used to refer to the experience of a person with dementia (see Scottish Government 2015) during an episode of 'challenging behaviour'. The British Psychological Society (2018) used the term 'Behaviour that Challenges' (BtC), taken from the first British NICE-SCIE Dementia Guideline 42 (2007, p.210), to include distress in both the person with a dementia and/or the carer(s). Thus, the person with dementia may or may not show distress, but the carer (or others interacting with the person) may find their dementia-related behavioural changes distressing. Bio-medical constructs of these dementia-related behavioural challenges include Neuropsychiatric Symptoms, Behavioural and Psychological Symptoms in Dementia (BPSD), or more recently 'Non-Cognitive Symptoms' (NICE 2018). The burden of these symptoms remains the most costly personal and economic aspects of dementia particularly for family carers. In practice, support for reducing distress associated with the challenges of dementia symptoms requires the practitioner to consider the interplay of interactions between the person and their family carer (Song *et al.* 2018), who if the terms 'informal' or 'unpaid' carer is used may also include friends or others in the social network.

This chapter outlines recent evidence for supporting family carers and reports on a short-term structured group intervention for family carers of people with mild dementia living at home in Norway.

Effective interventions

Tailored multicomponent psychosocial interventions are promising types of interventions in reducing the challenges encountered by family carers. The strongest evidence comes from case-specific structured support protocols targeting unmet health and psychosocial need in the person with dementia. These are described by reviewers in various ways, including individual formulation approach for analysing and managing challenging behaviours (Holle *et al.* 2016), Describe, Investigate, Create, Evaluate – the DICE approach (Kales, Gitlin and Lyketsos 2015), a step-by-step method to manage behavioural symptoms in dementia – and functional-analysis-based interventions (Dyer *et al.* 2018; Moniz-Cook *et al.* 2012; Moniz-Cook *et al.* 2017). Successful individualised interventions appear to require components tailored to both the person with dementia and the carer, delivered over a time of up-to six months, with periodic review (Brodaty and Arasaratnam 2012). The most common interventions for carers include helping them use psycho-education problem-solving methods, skills training (such as behaviour management strategies, communication skills training), self-care (such as health management, stress management and counselling), activity planning and enhancing social support (Brodaty and Arasaratnam 2012). Among researchers and practitioners there is much agreement that it is important to specifically attend to family carers' needs.

Distress can arise from perceived relationship changes and unmet carer needs. In Norway we found that experiences of loss and loneliness, role change and communication alteration balanced against their coping resources, are all part of carers' needs for support (Bjørge, Sæteren and Ulstein 2019). Feast *et al.* (2016a, 2016b) have outlined the significant unmet emotional needs of carers who support their relatives, and how psychosocial factors such as guilt, burden and a carer's own reaction can affect distress. Parkinson *et al.* (2017) identified five key themes emerging from their review of what works for carers:

- extending social assets
- strengthening psychological resources
- maintaining physical health
- safeguarding quality of life
- ensuring timely availability of external resources.

They conclude that these five factors interact to provide the support that bolsters carer 'resilience' and sustains family care. Gaugler, Reese and Mittelman (2018) described the findings and translations into practice of the landmark 'family counselling' New York University Caregiver Intervention (NYUIC) of over two and half decades. This early work reduced spouse-carer stress and depression; it also improved their health and delayed breakdown of care at home. Their recent work with carers describes the heterogeneity of perceived helpfulness of the family counselling programme: support groups were reported as helpful for managing parents' behavioural challenges; counselling for coping with emotional problems; both counselling and support groups for finding additional assistance; and support groups for managing functional problems and ongoing changes that occurred. In England the eight-week multicomponent individual psychological therapy for family carers START (STrAtegies for RelaTives) improved coping and mood disorders in the carer (Li *et al.* 2014). Some carers continued to use methods from START for over two years, with helpful components reported as: relaxation techniques, dementia education, strategies to help manage behaviour, contact with the therapist, and changing unhelpful thoughts (Sommerlad *et al.* 2014).

Most successful interventions have involved highly qualified therapists, such as psychologists and other health professionals, and can therefore be expensive. In Norwegian municipalities most health workers supporting people with dementia and their carer(s) are either nurses or nurse assistants, while in the UK most care workers, while often very skilled, have little training, there is high staff turnover and sickness, and many are low paid. Currently, with an increased focus on family carers' importance in postponing unwanted moves to care homes and on the need to support care workers to be effective and to want to stay in their jobs, effective short-term programmes for carers and care workers are needed to support them. However, we also need to better understand the characteristics of those who benefit from such approaches and those who do not. This does not ignore the wider contexts of low pay and low status for care workers but serves to enhance their working lives. It also does not ignore the widespread lack of recognition and support for carers in society.

The Norwegian group intervention
Design and description

This one-year randomised controlled trial recruited 171 people with dementia with their carers from seven Norwegian memory clinics (Ulstein *et al.* 2007a). Carers participated in either a short-term group-based intervention in addition to standard six-month follow-up or received 'treatment as usual', consisting of standard six-month follow-up at the memory clinic. General assistance from the memory clinic staff was offered to both groups.

The intervention lasted for four-and-a-half months, consisting of seven group sessions (Table 11.1). It began with three hours of education about dementia, provided by a geriatrician or psychiatrist, followed by six closed group meetings of six to eight carers. These two-hour sessions were facilitated by one leader. Structured problem solving was used to discuss carers' everyday dementia-care-related problems. The first three group sessions occurred fortnightly to foster group cohesiveness, followed by four sessions every third to fourth week, to give carers time to try out new solutions. Usually, two different problems were discussed during a session where common problems included the management of everyday behavioural or emotional symptoms, eliciting help from other family members or others, and encouraging the person with dementia to accept help. Structured agenda-based meetings (Table 11.1) started with a few minutes of 'small talk', then focused on reviewing the problem discussed at the last meeting (including examining solutions that hadn't worked), then new specific problem(s) were prioritised from the range of problems that carers said they were struggling with.

Table 11.1: Study design and methods

	Week 0	Week 2	Week 4	Week 7	Week 10	Week 14	Week 18	4.5 months	12 months
	Seminar	Six group sessions with six to eight participants							
Intervention – baseline	**Education about:** Dementia in general Dementia symptoms Pharmacological treatment Psychosocial treatment Introduction of problem-solving	Structured problem-solving: 1. Definition of a problem (as concrete as possible) 2. Brainstorming: all proposals were recorded on a flipchart 3. Discussing the proposed solutions – pros and cons 4. Choosing a solution or a combination of solutions 5. Detailed preparations for how to carry out the chosen solution 6. Evaluation at the next meeting						Retesting of carers	Retesting of patients and carers
Control – baseline	People with dementia and carers – 'treatment as usual'							Retesting of carers	Retesting of patients and carers

Delivery of the intervention: The group leader

To deliver the intervention the group leader used both practical tasks and therapeutic skills.

Practical tasks included:

- Preparing the group room with equipment (table, chairs and flipchart).

- Planning the seating arrangements to ensure maximum participation from everyone attending. We learned that seating in low chairs around a coffee table or an oblong table with the leader seated at one end, increased the potential of two carers inadvertently joining forces to talk throughout whilst others then remained silent. In another group, the only male carer took the chair that was at the end of the table and soon took over the group. For the next session, since he was the only one drinking tea, the group leader placed his tea cup in an alternative position thus allowing her to manage the problem-solving activity. These examples show the importance of planning environmental details like the type of table and seating arrangements. We concluded that a round or square table worked best to promote the group leader's face-to-face contact with the participants.

- Agenda setting and time-keeping.

- Monitoring the discussion to ensure its relevance to most carers.

Therapeutic skills included:

- Good knowledge of dementia and group dynamics to prevent isolation of any one group member. This often involved formulating similar situations facing at least two carers and actively pinpointing these, instead of focusing on differences, to promote a sense of group cohesion.

- Active listening and summarising skills to pinpoint a problem that was relevant to the majority of carers at a given time, since often only one or two carers were able to specify a problem to be resolved, so engaging the other carers was a challenge – for example: *'Even though the situations you are telling about are different, it seems to me that you all are expressing a need to be relieved, but are struggling with how to make your family member accept the help offered. Perhaps we can start with Maja [pseudonym] and see how she can deal with her husband's reluctance to visit the day-centre?'*

- Reformulating a problem in as concrete a way as possible, since often problems discussed were vaguely expressed and could undermine solutions that could be implemented.

- Reaching solutions by:

  – first collecting ideas from the group, writing out all suggestions on a flipchart (even ones that might be difficult to implement) so for example if the carer said: *'I have tried that and it didn't work out'* or *'I could never imagine doing that'*, the leader would open the discussion up further with comments such as *'Sure… but let us write it up, as others in the group may find the proposal helpful'*

  – then asking the person who raised the problem to consider the advantages and disadvantages of each proposal.

Finally, the leader and group helped with the choice of solution(s) to be tried out and facilitated discussion on how to implement this, including, if relevant, considering practical matters such as who to contact, where to find telephone numbers, and when the carer might try the chosen solution(s). Often suggestions had not worked because there had been insufficient exploration of the problem at the time or not enough planning of how the carer could carry out the chosen strategy. The availability of two group leaders would have allowed one to lead on problem-solving while the other held responsibility for writing up solutions and ensuring that all participants were given the opportunity to contribute.

Outcomes
Distress
The Neuropsychiatric Inventory (NPI: Cummings 1997) to measure neuropsychiatric symptoms and the Relatives' Stress Scale (RSS: Greene *et al.* 1982) to measure distress (referred to here as 'burden') were primary outcome measures (Ulstein *et al.* 2007b). Burden

increased in both intervention and control groups. However more carers in the control group moved from 'the low burden group (RSS < 23)' to a medium or high burden group, after 4.5 months compared to the intervention group. Detailed subgroup analysis showed a statistically significant difference in neuropsychiatric symptoms (NPI score) in favour of the intervention group among women with dementia compared with women with dementia in the control group. Explanations for these findings are: first, that carers of women with dementia were predominantly husbands and adult children with a different caring approach compared with wife carers, who constituted the majority supporters of men with dementia; second, husbands may have perceived their caring tasks as 'meaningful' whilst adult children often had to organise help from other family members and the municipality (these tensions were often discussed in groups); third, the more distressed wives may not have taken up educational problem-solving strategies as fully as husbands and adult children – the latter groups may have developed more realistic expectations thus enabling them to put what they learned into practice.

Although distressing symptoms were important contributors to the burden of care (Ulstein *et al.* 2007b), the increase in these among women with dementia in the control group was not followed by an increase in their burden scores. This demonstrates that burden (carer distress) is not always directly related to reported symptoms, confirming opinion that improving the experiences of carers can be a legitimate target of interventions (Bird and Moniz-Cook 2008). This study also demonstrates that not all carers are the same – there may be gender-related carer roles and needs (e.g. task-orientated problem-solving approaches versus emotional nurture) and the meaning of distress (Bjørge *et al.* 2019; Feast *et al.* 2016a), and its impact may differ across spouses/partners and adult children.

Carer experiences – 'being in the same boat'

Most carers appeared to find the number of sessions sufficient. Some were reluctant to accept the group approach; however, the benefits of taking part in group sessions with other carers were reported by many:

- sharing the emotional challenges of having a close family member with dementia

- sharing the psychological processes of grief and losses associated with dementia

- sharing tips and experiences on how to deal with dementia symptoms so that they become easier to live with

- finding the right level of care for both the person with dementia and the family at the right time.

The following comments[1] highlight the importance of peer support thorough meeting other carers and exchanging experiences, and also the spin-off for the group leader.

Dag, a husband stated:

> 'I was reluctant to apply for a daycare centre for my wife, but hearing the two siblings in the group telling about their positive experiences with their mother's daycare centre, gave me courage to apply for my wife. Now in retrospect, I feel ashamed that I held back, as I see that she has got a much better quality of life!'

Carers also discussed doing practical things together with the family member with dementia, and simultaneously dealing with conflicting emotions like love, joy, sorrow and anger.

Astrid, a daughter, said:

> 'I thought it was something wrong with me, that I was about to get crazy due to all the allegations and suspicions my mother directed to me when I was helping her with practical tasks she didn't master, especially as she was just kind and decent when she was with other people. Then I learned that others in the group had experienced the same, and it was easier for me to lean back telling myself that it was the illness...'

Annette, a group leader, noted that:

> 'Through this study I learned to trust the carers and give the participants the opportunity of finding their own solutions, in other words, working with the "hands on the back", not give advice!'

---

1   All names of participants in this chapter are pseudonyms.

Reflections: What might work for whom

There was wide variation among participants, such as their relationship, age, levels of stress and reports of distress. This had implications for working with a group within a randomised controlled study design where it was not possible to balance groups by participants' gender, age and relationship with their relative. The majority of carers in this study said that they had learned a lot from other group members. For example, Erik whose mother had dementia, and who joined the group along with his father, said:

> 'Through participating in the group I have a much better understanding of my father's situation. We have subsequently been able to allocate tasks in a better way.'

However, levels of burden and experiences of distress need be taken into account for an intervention such as this. Wife carers were overrepresented in the study and reported higher levels of burden, emotional distress and negative feelings towards the person with dementia than husband carers (Ulstein *et al.* 2007b). The intervention had no impact on carers who were very stressed (i.e. > 30 points on the RSS). There were qualitative observations that some were too upset to engage in problem solving, tending to monopolise discussions by repeating their difficulties in group meetings but appearing unable to try out suggestions that were made to manage their problem. They may have benefited from individualised counselling and emotional support to help them manage life with their relative, perhaps followed by attendance at a peer support group. Some carers appeared to have misunderstood the meaning of their relatives' behaviour. For example: Mrs C tells the group that her husband continues to drive even though he has no valid driver's licence (the *situation*). She was then asked by the leader if she had any *theories* about why he would do so. Mrs C replied: *'He is doing it to annoy me.'*

In some cases, with a discussion such as this, group members may have been able to help the carer attribute the situation to dementia, but in other cases the carer might benefit from an individually formulated functional-analytic approach to help them understand the multifactorial cause(s) of their relatives' behaviour (Dyer *et al.* 2018; Holle *et al.* 2016; Moniz-Cook *et al.* 2012, 2017).

Summary

This was a short-term psychosocial intervention programme for family carers that included (a) dementia education to improve understanding of how dementia symptoms affect behaviour and emotions, and (b) structured problem solving. It identified the characteristics of the carers and people with dementia that responded positively and those for whom the intervention was perhaps premature or not so effective. It provides good evidence of the need to address carers' heterogeneity – not all interventions will work for all carers. Findings indicate that gender, kinship, the level of burden of care and levels of distress have to be taken into account when implementing interventions for carers. Education and problem solving may be more beneficial for non-spouses/partners (adult children) and some husbands, but more distressed carers, especially wives, may benefit more from an individualised approach. We also need evidence of what works with same-sex partners.

There is a continuing need to recognise carers as partners in care but also to respond to differences between carers and to have a range of effective options. Evidence-based interventions to support family carers are hard to put into practice (Dickinson *et al.* 2017). Therefore, working with carers who support a close family member with dementia will require skills that could be encouraged by educators and by experienced practitioners to foster capacity and confidence in managing the everyday problems that arise.

References

Bird, M. and Moniz-Cook, E. (2008) 'Challenging Behaviour in Dementia: A Psychosocial Approach to Intervention.' In B. Woods and L. Clare (eds) *Handbook of the Clinical Psychology of Ageing* (Chapter 33, pp.571–596). Chichester: John Wiley & Sons.

Bjørge, H., Sæteren, B. and Ulstein, I. D. (2019) 'Experience of companionship among family caregivers of persons with dementia: A qualitative study.' *Dementia 18*, 1, 228–244.

British Psychological Society (2018) *Evidence briefing: 'Behaviour that challenges' in dementia.* Accessed on 2/4/2019 at www.bps.org.uk/sites/bps.org.uk/files/Policy/Policy%20-%20Files/Evidence%20briefing%20-%20behaviour%20that%20challenges%20in%20dementia.pdf

Brodaty, H. and Arasaratnam, C. (2012) 'Meta-analysis of nonpharmacological interventions for neuropsychiatric symptoms of dementia.' *American Journal of Psychiatry 169*, 946–953.

Cummings, J.L. (1997) 'The Neuropsychiatric Inventory: Assessing psychopathology in dementia patients.' *Neurology 48*, 10–16.

Dickinson, C., Dow, J., Gibson, G., Hayes, L., Robalino, S. and Robinson, L. (2017) 'Psychosocial intervention for carers of people with dementia: What components are most effective and when? A systematic review of systematic reviews.' *International Psychogeriatric, 29*, 1, 31–43.

Dyer, S.M., Harrison, S.L., Laver, K.E., Whitehead, C. and Crotty, M. (2018) 'An overview of systematic reviews of pharmacological and non-pharmacological interventions for the treatment of behavioral and psychological symptoms of dementia.' *International Psychogeriatrics 30*, 3, 295–309.

Feast, A., Orrell, M., Charlesworth, G., Melunsky, N., Poland, F. and Moniz-Cook, E. (2016a) 'Behavioural and Psychological Symptoms in Dementia (BPSD) and the challenges for family carers: A systematic review.' *British Journal of Psychiatry 208*, 5, 429–434.

Feast, A., Moniz-Cook, E., Stoner, C., Charlesworth, G. and Orrell, M. (2016b) 'A systematic review of the relationship between Behavioural and Psychological Symptoms (BPSD) and caregiver wellbeing.' *International Psychogeriatrics 28*, 11, 1761–1774.

Gaugler, J., Reese, M. and Mittelman, M.S. (2018) 'Process Evaluation of the NYU Caregiver Intervention – Adult Child.' *The Gerontologist 58*, 2, e107–e117.

Greene, J.G., Smith, R., Gardiner, M. and Timbur, G.C. (1982) 'Measuring behavioural disturbance of elderly demented patients in the community and its effects on relatives: A factor analytic study.' *Age and Ageing 11*, 121–126.

Holle, D., Halek, M., Holle B. and Pinkert, C. (2016) 'Individualized formulation-led interventions for analyzing and managing challenging behavior of people with dementia – an integrative review.' *Ageing and Mental Health 21*, 12, 1229–1247.

Kales, H.C., Gitlin, L N. and Lyketsos, C.G. (2015) 'State of the art review: Assessment and management of behavioral and psychological symptoms of dementia.' *British Medical Journal 350*, h369.

Li, R., Cooper, C., Barber, J., Rapaport, P. Griffin, M. and Livingston, G. (2014) 'Coping strategies as mediators of the effect of the START (strategies for RelaTives) intervention on psychological morbidity for family carers of people with dementia in a randomised controlled trial.' *Journal of Affective Disorders 168*, 298–305.

Moniz-Cook, E.D., Swift, K., James, I., Malouf, R., De Vugt, M. and Verhey, F. (2012) *Functional analysis-based interventions for challenging behaviour in dementia (review).* The Cochrane Library, Issue 2.

Moniz-Cook, E., Hart, C., Woods, B., Whitaker, C. *et al.* (2017) *Challenge Demcare: Management of Challenging Behaviour in Dementia at Home and in Care Homes.* Southampton, NIHR.

National Institute for Health and Clinical Excellence/Social Care Institute for Excellence (2007) *Dementia: Supporting People with Dementia and their Carers in Health and Social Care.* NICE clinical guideline NG42. London: NICE.

National Institute for Health and Care Excellence (NICE) (2018) *Dementia – Assessment, Management and Support for People Living with Dementia and Their Carers.* NICE Clinical Guideline NG97. Accessed on 3/8/2018 at www.nice.org.uk/guidance/ng97

Parkinson, M., Carr, S.M., Rushmer, R. and Abley, C. (2017) 'Investigating what works to support family carers of people with dementia: A rapid realist review.' *Journal of Public Health 39*, 4, e290–e301

Scottish Government (2015) *Quality and Excellence in Specialist Dementia Care (QESDC): Baseline One-off Self-assessment Tool and Reporting Arrangements.* Accessed on 1/4/2019 at www.gov.scot/publications/quality-excellence-specialist-dementia-care-qesdc-baseline-one-self-assessment-tool-reporting-arrangements/pages/14

Song, J.A., Park, M., Park, J., Cheon, H.J. and Lee, M. (2018) 'Patient and caregiver interplay in behavioral and psychological symptoms of dementia: Family caregivers' experience.' *Clinical Nursing Research 27*, 1, 12–34.

Sommerlad, A., Manela, M., Cooper, C., Rapaport, P. and Livingston, G. (2014) 'START (STrAtegies for RelaTives) coping strategy for family carers of adults with dementia:

Qualitative study of participants' views about the intervention.' *British Medical Journal Open 4*, e005273.

Ulstein, I.D., Sandvik, L., Wyller, T.B. and Engedal, K. (2007a) 'A one-year randomized controlled psychosocial intervention study among family carers of dementia patients – effects on patients and carers.' *Dementia Geriatric Cognitive Disorders 24*, 6, 469–475.

Ulstein, I., Bruun Wyller, T. and Engedal, K. (2007b) 'The Relative Stress Scale: A useful instrument to identify various aspects of carer burden in dementia.' *International Journal of Geriatric Psychiatry 22* 1, 61–67.

Chapter 12

Supporting People with Dementia Through Music

Alfredo Raglio, Maria Gianelli, Esme Moniz-Cook and Jill Manthorpe

Introduction

Music and music-based therapeutic interventions range from music therapy provided by skilled therapists to engaging in musical activities. They can include active music therapy taking psychological and rehabilitative approaches, active music therapy with people with dementia and families, 'music-based interventions', singing during care provision, and listening to music and background music (Raglio *et al.* 2014). These can be part of a bundle of psychosocial interventions in dementia care since there is good evidence that, at least in the short term, they can help reduce neuropsychiatric symptoms (McDermott *et al.* 2013; van der Steen *et al.* 2018). Indeed a systematic review on therapies for neuropsychiatric symptoms, (also known as Behavioural and Psychological Symptoms of Dementia – BPSD, or behavioural symptoms that cause distress) identified music therapy as the most common non-pharmacological therapy that has been studied; followed by aromatherapy and massage, laughter, structured activities, animal-assisted interventions, environmental interventions, simulated presence, dance movement, art and combination therapies (Olley and Morales 2017).

The seminal music therapy studies were conducted in care homes in Italy, where small-group music therapy was reported to reduce neuropsychiatric symptoms, with additional observed positive effect of the therapist–resident social relationship during the course of therapy, irrespective of the severity of dementia (Raglio *et al.* 2008, 2010a, 2010b, 2012, 2015). The first of these also noted some positive effects lasting to follow-up (Raglio *et al.* 2008). Reviews by examining various aspects of the value of music for people with dementia continue to emerge (Aleixo, Santos and Dourado 2017; Chang *et al.* 2015; Elliott and Gardner 2018; McDermott *et al.* 2013; Meyer and O'Keefe 2018; Raglio *et al.* 2014; Särkämö 2018), as do new randomised controlled trials (RCTs) in care homes, such as those of Ho *et al.* (2018) and Cheung, Lai and Wong (2018). However, in many countries the potential of music in the care of people with dementia is not fully recognised. McDermott *et al.* (2013) note that '[i]t is only when the study findings are implemented in practice, that the potential long-term effects of an intervention become beneficial for people with dementia' (p.793).

The term *music-based therapeutic interventions* is used in research on biopsychosocial approaches in dementia care (Raglio *et al.* 2014; Särkämö 2018). However, music therapy activities are frequently referred to in a less technical sense as *general music sessions*, taking place in health or care settings, in care practice or general daily activity. Many practitioners will be aware of the different uses of sound and music but not always their possible specific, *intentional* use for therapeutic or care purposes. This chapter reports practice developments in care homes bringing music to the lives of residents and staff. It argues that seeing music as a participatory art (Zeelig, Killick and Fox 2014) may be a positive new direction for care home practice in particular. It also outlines the potential for adopting or commissioning music-based approaches with people with dementia, since the use of music in care settings can be an enjoyable activity for residents, their visitors and members of staff alike.

Music and music therapy

The term *music-based therapeutic interventions* was recently used in a review of the evidence (van der Steen *et al.* 2018), while others describe *specialist music therapy,* defined as a special form of psychotherapy (Gold *et al.* 2009; Raglio 2011). In this form of therapy, the *relational process* set in motion between person with dementia and therapist is the core of the whole therapeutic activity. The profession of music therapy claims that, by its very nature, it is person-centred: because at the heart of the experience is the relationship between the music therapist and their recognition of the person with dementia, with their personal biography or life history, personality, likes and dislikes, as well as the type and degree of neurological impairment taken into account. Such an approach helps us think about music as more than the playing of background music or occasional singing – but should not exclude these aspects of music in the environment. The potential of using music in many care settings may be under-used.

In person-centred care 'all actions are seen as meaningful' (Kitwood 1997), therefore an underlying principle of person-centred care is that the actions of the person with dementia are messages that the individual is attempting to communicate: as such, they might be seen as 'mysteries' to be explored and possibly 'solved' by the person and those supporting them together. Since person-centred care is achieved by recognising the person that exists beyond the deteriorating cognitive state of dementia and how they are expressing themselves at the time of care, one form of self-enhancing music-based practice is musical improvisation or making music. This active approach to music is a non-verbal strategy that partly by-passes the cognitive component and addresses the person directly, involving them in a emotional-relational event. A therapeutic encounter takes place in this relational context, which often relies on musical sounds rather than singing. By concentrating on sound as a means of communication it is possible, even with a person with severe dementia who is no longer able to speak, to build alternative channels of communication with the person instead of conversation (Raglio 2010). Thus, music-based interventions may be an approach worth considering when other approaches do not seem to be working, such as talking or touching. A relationship can be built from enjoyment of sound 'in the moment'.

The evidence base

To explore the extensive evidence base of effectiveness of music interventions in dementia, we refer particularly to the most recent Cochrane review, whilst noting that most reviews conclude that 'more research is needed'.

This review (van der Steen et al. 2018) of what they termed 'treatments' based on music was conducted to see whether such treatments improved the emotional wellbeing and quality of life of people with dementia. All eligible studies had taken place with care home residents and the interventions (treatments) had to involve at least five sessions. The Cochrane reviewers searched for evidence about their effects on emotional, behavioural, social or cognitive (e.g. thinking and remembering) problems in people with dementia. The outcomes investigated included alterations in quality of life, mood disturbance (such as depression and anxiety), behavioural problems, aspects of social behaviour and cognition following the therapy sessions. The authors conclude:

> Providing people with dementia who are in institutional care with at least five sessions of a music-based therapeutic intervention probably reduces depressive symptoms and improves overall behavioural problems at the end of treatment. It may also improve emotional well-being and quality of life and reduce anxiety, but may have little or no effect on agitation or aggression or on cognition. We are uncertain about effects on social behaviour, and about long-term effects. (van der Steen *et al.* 2018, p.4)

Texts exist outlining a rationale and guidance for clinical application of the evidence for music therapy (Raglio 2010). However, there is also new interest in the positive outcomes of music system-wide in care homes rather than searching for outcomes that address only neuropsychiatric symptoms that cause challenges and distress. For example, McDermott, Orrell and Ridder (2014a) found that music can support the personal psychology of people with dementia and the social psychology of the care home environment, concluding that the effects of music go beyond the reduction of distressing symptoms. Their study included both care home staff and residents.

What is needed for general musical activities?

The enjoyment of music can be fostered also by family carers and care workers. In these instances, interventions are led by someone without specific training and are mainly based on a culture of care that values residents' wellbeing and enables staff to work with residents rather than focusing on simply completing their tasks. The work of activity coordinators, care home staff with specific responsibilities for individual and group activities in care homes, often extends to bringing music into the life of a care home (see the work of the NAPA – the National Activity Providers Association[1]) and to helping people living

---

1   https://napa-activities.co.uk

in care homes participate in the wider community through taking part in activities such as attending musical events.

> **Ideas adapted from NAPA about organising singing activities**
> Arrange a series of short singing sessions with your local community connections.
>
> Be innovative about where and how this might happen. Perhaps you could take residents to the local senior school or college rather than have them visit you? Of course you can stay in your home and invite lots of different groups in.
>
> Connect with the community in public settings. Could you sing in the local bandstand, on the beach or in the shopping centre?
>
> Get local people to join in and support your singing.
>
> Choose a few songs that your residents really enjoy singing, but please make sure they are from the 1950s onwards.
>
> Print lots of large-print song sheets to hand out.

Therapeutic interventions are based upon specific, mostly active, techniques (*active* music therapy), where more general musical encounters aim to stimulate communication and relationships and the sharing of feelings. This is what produces the character of the intervention, whatever the model or the contents of the activity might be. In addition, *music listening* approaches (see Massaia *et al.* 2018) may be employed, based not just on listening to the music, but on the possibility that someone starts speaking or singing or making noises suggesting pleasure or enjoyment following hearing the music.

This shifts attention from a specifically therapeutic component, allowing for the suggestion that sound and music themselves might exert positive effects, such as producing wellbeing, stimulating liveliness and promoting socialisation. Several music-based interventions in care homes for people with dementia may be arranged to counter apparent symptoms of apathy or low mood or simply to provide an atmosphere of wellbeing. Such interventions include making music with residents, usually in groups, inviting them to accompany live or recorded pieces of music with or without a musical instrument, by freely making use of song, body movements, rhythmical tapping, and so on. In other instances, residents listen to music that may trigger memories, or promote another response from the person with dementia or prompt general relaxation.

Most people with dementia appear to prefer to listen to well-known music or rhythmic pieces, since these seem more likely to stimulate them, rather than to simply reduce tension. Some musical activity can be more purposeful, and may be tailored to the person's needs or preferences: for example, the care worker or family member selects a playlist containing the person's favourite music and uses it at specific moments of the day. The pieces chosen are the result of taking a music history from the resident where possible, finding out what they like or dislike (see the Playlist for Life initiative in Case Study 12.1), in addition to information about the person's life story and personality, collected in conversations with family members, care workers and, whenever possible, the person themselves.

Case Study 12.1 – Harry and Margaret

Harry and Margaret were the first couple that Playlist for Life worked with. Harry had severe dementia and lived in a care home. Margaret, his wife, came every day to see him and left most days in tears. Harry had stopped responding to her. A video clip captures what happened when they started listening to his playlist together.[2]

Yet another approach, applied almost instinctively when relating to people with dementia, is the use of singing. Addressing the person with dementia through singing can facilitate contact, thus enabling the person to become more open to friendly approaches and to interaction. The systematic application of this approach by care home workers, may be useful when undertaking tasks such as washing or bathing (Hammar *et al.* 2011), medication administration, moving and handling, and so on.

In other examples of music-based activities in care homes (Case Study 12.2), visiting professional musicians may provide stimulating activity, but such one-off or irregular activities are not easy to capture in effectiveness research. Nonetheless, many such examples of positive outcomes are reported in the media and some appear to be almost

---

2 See www.playlistforlife.org.uk/Blog/harry-margarets-story

transformational in the eyes of family members. Harm is rarely reported. What we may conclude is a need for a greater individualisation (personalisation) of these interventions, almost regardless of the techniques employed.

Case Study 12.2 – **John and his daughter Linda** (Live Music Now)[3]

Diagnosed with mixed dementia some ten years ago, John, aged 82, has suffered many losses in recent years – losing his wife and then his son soon afterwards. He moved to a care home to be closer to his daughter, Linda. She says he is finding it difficult to make friends and is reluctant to join in activities, choosing instead to remain in his room for most of the day.

In August 2016, John began taking part in music sessions with Live Music Now musicians Joe and Jess at Sabrina House as part of the New Age Music project. The care home staff quickly saw how John engaged with the music, singing along and playing percussion instruments. They mentioned this to Linda, who regularly visits her father.

Linda found reports of singing difficult to believe. She had never once heard her father sing, not even 'Happy Birthday'. Linda was able to go along to one of the sessions and hearing her father sing for the first time was a very emotional experience for her. She says it gave them a connection that she hadn't felt before. John also experiences severe anxiety attacks, usually occurring two or three times during a typical visit. On the days where John had taken part in the music sessions Linda noted that he didn't experience any panic attacks.

Personalisation can also affect care practice. There are many examples of how music can augment the care home worker's repertoire. These include research investigating the positive potential for care workers to sing during activities that the resident with dementia finds distressing (Livingston *et al.* 2005), as reported above, and encouragement of positive musical encounters between a family member and the resident with dementia.

---

3 Adapted from www.livemusicnow.org.uk/case_studies/title/New-Age-Music-in-Shropshire-John-s-Story/item/69435

Everyday digital opportunities

The use of everyday technology is something that can be used to personalise care, with the availability of access to music from previous decades or organised in themes and by images. The BBC RemArc archive was created in conjunction with the UK Alzheimer's Society, and researchers from Dundee University and St Andrews University. This resource can be used on handheld tablets and needs little setting up or technological skill. See: https:// remarc.bbcrewind.co.uk and https://bbcnewslabs.co.uk/projects/ bbc-rewind

With reference to listening to music, there appears to be a consensus that being able to listen to a favourite piece of music or at least familiar music contributes to the person with dementia's quality of life. If the music has some emotional meaning for the person with dementia, because it is linked to their biography or personality and characteristics, this may contribute to the building up of a positive, secure atmosphere. In turn this may reduce possibly distressing symptoms of dementia such as anxiety, agitation and depression. Personalisation, of course, is needed to respect the fact that not everyone may like music or certain types of music – and that preferences may change. The development of questionnaires to assess an individual's interest in music interest, specifically for use in people with dementia, was undertaken by McDermott *et al.* (2014b) whose Music in Dementia Assessment Scales (MiDAS) can be used to measure engagement with music and to provide insight into who might be likely to respond well to musical activities.

Background music appears to be sometimes effective, for example in nursing homes (Hicks-Moore 2005), but in practice it would be appropriate to consult about this if it is being mooted as well as to pilot such an initiative.

Discussion

Despite the many aspects still needing clarification and more in-depth examination, a good deal of evidence is now apparent, with consequently important implications and indications for care. Many studies of music therapy with people with dementia have focused on reducing distressing or challenging behaviour, whereas studies related to the possible efficacy of sound and music upon cognitive and physiological/neural aspects are only just emerging (see Raglio *et al.* 2010b; Särkämö 2018; Särkämö *et al.* 2014). Case studies run the risk of bias in presenting generally positive accounts of interventions but can be useful in conveying the importance of creativity and encouraging personalised approaches to care. Until recently, relevant outcome measures for studies that target the full range of aims of music-based interventions have not been available but more are emerging (see, e.g., MiDAS: McDermott *et al.* 2014b in care homes; and Tan *et al.* 2019 in an acute hospital).

One point that is highly relevant to care home settings is that a direct therapist–person-with-dementia interaction – subject to a prior assessment of the person's suitability for this kind of intervention – might have greater efficacy than a group intervention. However many people with dementia living in care homes will be taking part in musical activities in a group, guided by care workers or volunteers with some musical skills. Others may encounter music in the course of personal care (Hammar *et al.* 2011) or at times of distress. Zeelig *et al.* (2014) comment that 'the arts are effective at alleviating boundaries between service providers and people with dementia and in providing new insights for the dementia workforce and family members' (p.24).

The future

It remains curious that, while music as a psychosocial intervention has been widely studied, for practitioners working in care homes the evidence often appears uncertain and only of remote application (for an example of the translation of a music therapist's expertise to the world of care see Rio 2009). Most studies call for further research. We do have some ideas of what should be the priority areas for research, and perhaps time is needed to consider these and to concentrate not only on therapy but also on enhancing wellbeing and compassionate care. Ridder (2016) suggests that greater attention should be given to age, gender, ethnicity, cultural background and socio-economic status to consider equalities. She also recommends greater attention to technology, which, as this chapter has noted, is extending the repertoire of people supporting care home residents overall as well as those with dementia. Technology is potentially also enabling musical activities to be far more interactive. Finally, Ridder suggests that theory building would be a welcome addition to interdisciplinary work in this area.

Conclusions

Music has potential to enhance the lives of people with dementia, but perhaps more as a participatory art than has been generally realised. The evidence suggests that music-based interventions, in particular, as an activity aimed to reduce challenging symptoms causing distress or to improve relationships, can be undertaken with people with moderate-to-severe dementia. Some gains can be expected in care homes settings from both individual and small-group activities. Other musical activities can involve larger groups of people with dementia, with the aim of increasing socialisation and wellbeing. These community-based activities link with ideas of 'ageing in place' (Elliott and Gardner 2018), and many of them include people with dementia and their family members (Clark, Tamplin and Baker 2018), where longer-term benefits on some aspects of cognition and quality of life have been reported (Särkämö, *et al.* 2014).

Despite the interest in music in long-term settings, little research has been conducted on how to develop care home staff's skills in this area of practice and how to build on their creativity. We also need to move to broader implementation studies so that we can establish why some care homes and some staff appear to be able to offer music activities of all types to residents with evident enjoyment, while in others this seems more 'hit and miss' and depends on one individual's commitment or interest.

References

Aleixo, M., Santos, R. and Dourado, M. (2017) 'Efficacy of music therapy in the neuropsychiatric symptoms of dementia: Systematic review.' *Jornal Brasileiro de Psiquiatria 66,* 1, 52–61.

Chang, Y., Chu, H., Yang, C., Tsai, J. *et al.* (2015) 'The efficacy of music therapy for people with dementia: A meta-analysis of randomised controlled trials.' *Journal of Clinical Nursing 24,* 3425–3440.

Cheung, D., Lai, C. and Wong, F. (2018) 'Is music-with-movement intervention better than music listening and social activities in alleviating agitation of people with moderate dementia? A randomized controlled trial.' *Dementia. doi:*10.1177/1471301218800195

Clark, I., Tamplin, J. and Baker, F. (2018) 'Community-dwelling people living with dementia and their family caregivers experience enhanced relationships and feelings of wellbeing following therapeutic group singing: A qualitative thematic analysis.' *Frontiers in Psychology 9*, 1332.

Elliott, M. and Gardner, P. (2018) 'The role of music in the lives of older adults with dementia ageing in place: A scoping review.' *Dementia 17*, 2, 199–213.

Gold, C., Solli, H., Kroger V. and Lie S.A. (2009) 'Dose-response relationship in music therapy for people with serious mental disorders: Systematic review and meta-analysis.' *Clinical Psychology Review 293*, 19–207.

Hammar, L., Emami, A., Engström, G. and Götell, E. (2011) 'Communicating through caregiver singing during morning care situations in dementia care.' *Scandinavian Journal of Caring Sciences 25*, 1, 160–168.

Hicks-Moore, S. (2005) 'Relaxing music at mealtime in nursing homes.' *Journal of Gerontological Nursing, 31*, 12, 26–32.

Ho, R., Fong, T., Singh, C., Lee, P. *et al.* (2018) 'Managing behavioral and psychological symptoms in Chinese elderly with dementia via group-based music intervention: A cluster randomized controlled trial.' *Dementia.* doi:10.1177/1471301218760023

Kitwood, T. (1997) *Dementia Reconsidered: The Person Comes First.* Buckingham: Open University Press.

Livingston, G., Johnston, K., Katona, C., Paton, J., Lyketsos, C. and Old Age Task Force of the World Federation of Biological Psychiatry (2005) 'Systematic review of psychological approaches to the management of neuropsychiatric symptoms of dementia.' *American Journal of Psychiatry 162*, 11, 1996–2021.

Massaia, M., Reano, A., Luppi, C., Santagata, F., Marchetti, M. and Isaia, G. (2018) 'Receptive music interventions improve apathy and depression in elderly patients with dementia.' *Geriatric Care 4*, 7, 248.

McDermott, O., Crellin, N., Ridder, H. and Orrell, M. (2013) 'Music therapy in dementia: A narrative synthesis systematic review.' *International Journal of Geriatric Psychiatry 28*, 781–794.

McDermott, O., Orrell, M. and Ridder, H.M (2014a) 'The importance of music for people with dementia: The perspectives of people with dementia, family carers, staff and music therapists.' *Aging & Mental Health 18*, 6, 706–716.

McDermott, O., Orgeta, V., Ridder, H. and Orrell, M. (2014b) 'A preliminary psychometric evaluation of music in dementia assessment scales (MiDAS).' *International Psychogeriatrics 26*, 1011–1019.

Meyer, C. and O'Keefe, F. (2018) 'Non-pharmacological interventions for people with dementia: A review of reviews.' *Dementia.* doi:10.1177/1471301218813234

Olley, R. and Morales, A. (2017) 'Systematic review of evidence underpinning non-pharmacological therapies in dementia.' *Australian Health Review 42*, 4, 361–369.

Raglio, A. (2010) 'Music therapy and dementia.' *Non-Pharmacological Therapy in Dementia 1*, 1–14.

Raglio, A. (2011) 'When music becomes music therapy.' *Psychiatry and Clinical Neurosciences 65*, 7, 682–683.

Raglio, A., Bellelli, G., Traficante, D., Gianotti, M. *et al.* (2008) 'Efficacy of music therapy in the treatment of behavioral and psychiatric symptoms of dementia.' *Alzheimer Disease and Associated Disorders 22*, 2, 158–162.

Raglio, A., Bellelli, G., Traficante, D.,Gianotti, M. *et al.* (2010a) 'Efficacy of music therapy treatment based on cycles of sessions: A randomised controlled trial.' *Aging and Mental Health 14*, 8, 900–904.

Raglio, A., Oasi, O., Gianotti, M. and Manzoni, V. (2010b) 'Effects of music therapy on psychological symptoms and heart rate variability in patients with dementia: A pilot study.' *Current Aging Science 3*, 242–246.

Raglio, A., Bellelli, G., Traficante, D., Gianotti, M. *et al.* (2012) 'Addendum to "Efficacy of music therapy treatment based on cycles of sessions: A randomised controlled trial"'. *Aging Mental Health 16*, 2, 265–267.

Raglio, A., Filippi, S., Bellandi, D. and Stramba-Badiale, M. (2014) 'Global music approach to persons with dementia: Evidence and practice.' *Clinical interventions in Aging 9*, 1669–1676.

Raglio, A., Bellandi, D., Baiardi, P., Gianotti, M. *et al.* (2015) 'Effect of active music therapy and individualized listening to music on dementia: A multicenter randomized controlled trial.' *Journal of the American Geriatrics Society 63*, 8, 1534–1539.

Ridder, H. (2016) 'The Future of Music Therapy for Persons with Dementi.' In C. Dileo (ed.) *Envisioning the Future of Music Therapy* (pp.87–95). Philadelphia, PA: Temple University.

Rio, R. (2009) *Connecting through Music with People with Dementia: A Guide for Caregivers.* London: Jessica Kingsley Publishers.

Särkämö, T. (2018) 'Music for the ageing brain: Cognitive, emotional, social, and neural benefits of musical leisure activities in stroke and dementia.' *Dementia 17*, 6, 670–685.

Särkämö, T., Tervaniemi, M., Laitinen, S. and Numminen, A. (2014) 'Cognitive, emotional, and social benefits of regular musical activities in early dementia: Randomized controlled study.' *The Gerontologist, 54*, 4, 634–650.

Tan, J., Wee, S-L., Yeo, P., Choo, J., Ritholz, M. and Yap, P. (2019) 'A new music therapy engagement scale for persons with dementia.' *International Psychogeriatrics, 31*, 1, 49–58.

van der Steen, J., Smaling, H., van der Wouden, J., Bruinsma, M., Scholten, R. and Vink, A. (2018) 'Music-based therapeutic interventions for people with dementia.' *Cochrane Database of Systematic Reviews 7*, Art. No. CD003477.

Zeelig, H., Killik, J. and Fox, C. (2014) 'The participative arts for people living with a dementia: A critical review.' *International Journal of Ageing and Later Life 9*, 1, 7–34.

Related reading

Argyle, E. and Kelly, T. (2014) *Improving Quality of Life and End of Life Care for People with Dementia Using Personalised music: 'The Soundtrack to My Life' Tool.* Nottingham: University of Nottingham. http://eprints.nottingham.ac.uk/38699/1/UoN-Research-Document-Web-version.pdf

Kontas, P. and Grigorovich, A. (2018) 'Rethinking musicality in dementia as embodied and relational.' *Journal of Aging Studies.* doi:10.1016/j.jaging.2018.01.006

Raglio, A., Bellelli, G., Mazzola, P., Bellandi, D. et al. (2012) 'Music, music therapy and dementia: A review of literature and the recommendations of the Italian Psychogeriatric Association.' *Maturitas 72*, 4305–4310.

Chapter 13

Dancing with People
with Dementia

Iva Holmerová, Hana Vaňková, Michal Šteffl and Petr Veleta

Introduction

Dancing is a growing method used to engage people with dementia
in drawing on past interests though reminiscence (Coaten 2001) and
pleasurable activity (Guzman-Garcia, Hughes *et al.* 2013). Different
types of dance have been piloted with people who have a dementia, such
as: Latin dancing (Guzmán *et al.* 2016; Guzmán-Garcia, Mukaetova-
Ladinska and James 2013); waltzing, (O'Rourke *et al.* 2017; Rosler *et al.*
2002); Wu Tao dance therapy (Duignan, Hedley and Milverton 2009),
circle dancing (Hamill, Smith and Röhricht 2011) and salsa dancing
(Abreu and Hartley 2013). Many of these dance interventions aim
to reduce depression, agitation or distress in people with dementia
and/or carer burden, usually within a care home setting (Duignan *et al.*
2009; Hamill *et al.* 2011; O'Rourke *et al.* 2017). Duignan *et al.* (2009)
suggest that dance programmes may be particularly effective when
the spirits of both residents with dementia and staff in care homes are
enhanced by the activity. There are also descriptions of positive effects
on cognition, new skill learning and on everyday social functioning in
people with dementia (Christofoletti *et al.* 2008; Hokkanen *et al.* 2008;
Palo-Bengtsson and Ekman 2002; Rosler *et al.* 2002), and on leisure
activities between people with dementia and their families (Dupuis
et al. 2012; DiLauro *et al.* 2017). Some theorists connect body, mind
and dancing in dementia care using the notion of 'embodiment', which
here refers to the subjective sense of awareness in the person with
dementia, of their 'lived-body' experience of 'movement' (Coaten and
Newman-Bluestein 2013).

Dance in dementia is not often conceived as an exercise programme *per se*, but dance as an exercise with a relatively sedentary 84-year-old woman with Alzheimer's disease, who had multiple comorbidities and recurrent falls has been described (Abreu and Hartley 2013). The authors chose Salsa dancing since this was culturally familiar to the person with dementia, and report clinically meaningful improvements in a range of functions, such as strength mobility, gait distance and speed, with no reported falls at six-month follow-up. Many older people have movement impairments due to chronic conditions such as osteoporosis (bone weakening), osteopenia (low bone mass and strength) and sarcopenia (loss of muscle mass and strength), and associated reduced physical activity can have a negative impact on their mood (Vaňková *et al.* 2008).

Falls in older people have negative consequences, such as fracture, head injury and fears about falling, which restrict movement. Approaches aimed at preventing falls and their consequences in older people with and without dementia have become important, particularly for those living in care homes where the prevalence of these is high. A Cochrane review of interventions to prevent falls in community-dwelling older people (Gillespie *et al.* 2012), concluded that both group- and home-based personalised exercise programmes to enhance muscle strength and balance are effective. The authors noted that if systematic exercise programmes target more than one modality (including those that incorporate walking for those people who are sedentary), are planned properly and are carried out regularly, the risk of falls can reduce by half.

A second Cochrane review of programmes to prevent falls in hospitals and care homes was less conclusive (Cameron *et al.* 2012). The authors suggested that multimodal interventions in care facilities may be beneficial and could be the focus of future research. However, Hernandez *et al.* (2010) noted that many fall-prevention programmes do not enrol people with dementia, so less is known about benefits of fall-prevention interventions in dementia care. Notably, dementia itself is often accompanied by disturbances of movement and coordination, such as in the later stages of Alzheimer's disease (Jirák, Holmerová and Borzová 2009; Muir *et al.* 2013). In some cases, due to underlying pathology, movement difficulties may precede other dementia-related symptoms, as in Parkinson's related dementia.

Thus more evidence is required about how dance can help people with dementia to maintain strength and mobility to prevent the risks associated with falls. There are cautionary notes about group exercises that do not take account of individual needs and abilities where the risk of falling can be increased (Gillespie *et al.* 2012). Similarly, some cautionary notes are seen from the reminiscence-dance literature, where simply watching dancing was experienced positively by some people with dementia, but others had negative experiences of this (Ravelin, Isola and Kylmä 2013). Individualisation of multimodal exercise programmes is therefore a useful principle for dance-based interventions in older people with dementia.

Given that dancing may be a way to help with new learning in dementia (Rosler *et al.* 2002), it may suit many as an exercise programme. When tailored to an individual for both exercise and aspects of dance, it has scope to be both enjoyable and easy to engage with (Guzmán-Garcia *et al.* 2013; Hokkanen *et al.* 2008). It may also enhance cultural and emotional aspects that are important to wellbeing for some people (Abreu and Hartley 2013) and interpersonal contact and communication between people with dementia, family, friends and care practitioners (Palo-Bengtsson and Ekman 2002).

In this chapter we focus on enhancing movement in older people with dementia using dance as a means of 'exercise' particularly for those living in care homes. Our programme is set in the context of our previous work, taking an exercise perspective to dance, where benefits may occur through improved fitness of the lower limbs, which is an important factor in fall prevention (Holmerová *et al.* 2010), improved mood (Vaňková *et al.* 2014) and improved functioning (Machacova *et al.* 2017; Suchá and Holmerová 2016). First, we describe *EXDASE* (Exercise Dance for Seniors) our dance-based exercise intervention. Next we use our understanding of attitudes to exercise (Janeckova *et al.* 2013) and experience of *EXDASE* to outline key principles for implementation in care homes and other care settings.

Principles of EXDASE (Exercise Dance for Seniors)

This intervention is distinct from 'dance therapy', which requires a comprehensive therapeutic approach administered by a trained therapist. The recent Cochrane review on dance movement therapy in dementia included only interventions using trained therapists (Karkou and Meekums 2017). Notably, the authors were unable to find randomised controlled studies as most studies located did not use a trained therapist to deliver the intervention. In our group-based programme, a dancer or a dance instructor (who is not a therapist) prepares a dance-based exercise session. *EXDASE* uses the basic elements of movement based on the skills and capabilities of the participant. Exercises that promote balance, strength and fitness to promote overall physical condition and mood, as well as the prevention of sarcopenia and falls are usually important in most cases. A manual with guidance is available (see Veleta and Holmerová 2004). Key aspects of the programme are outlined below:

- Individualised exercise options are used to tailor care to the movement needs of a person with dementia, and the instructor then leads participants in the dance session.

- Assistants can be very helpful in larger groups or those with participants who have severe disabilities. Dance assistants may be staff or volunteers. Assistants not only help people with limited mobility but they are also actively involved in the *EXDASE* programme.

- Sessions are composed in such way that they are easy for people with dementia, but also accessible to other disabled people who may use different aids and assistive devices.

- It is very important during the session to recognise and appreciate the skills, achievements, contribution and creativity of all participants. For example, the dance instructor may say, 'It was so good to lift a leg like this. This is a real can-can' or, 'Oh yes, that hand movement was so graceful and elegant'.

- The session takes the form of dance, starting with communication, an invitation to dance and socialise, but it also includes practice elements of individualised exercise, focused on strength, balance, coordination and fitness and on harmonising the person's abilities and disabilities.

Description of the programme

The dancing session begins slowly with all participants seated on chairs in a circle. They then begin movements according to their individual abilities. The dance instructor prepares a simple choreography based on the movements of individual participants, and the group continues to exercise in a sitting position since this is thought to be easier than starting from a standing position (Stephan and Amthor 2011), although later they may progress to standing. Exercises include elements of fitness as well as strength and balance. The session ends with relaxation and a 'farewell', expressed both verbally and non-verbally. Throughout the session the emphasis is not only on physical exercise, but particularly also on communication, comfort and promoting a friendly group atmosphere.

In the initial phase, *EXDASE* participants, assistants and a dance instructor are seated in a circle. During this initial slow phase the dance instructor welcomes participants with a greeting and participants then greet each other, verbally and non-verbally. Next each person is invited to demonstrate or suggest 'their dance', with movements that they are able to perform. Factors to emphasise during the whole session are a sense of security, comfort and self-confidence. While seated, participants are able to concentrate on moving their head, trunk and limbs. During this initial warm-up phase participants 'offer' movements to demonstrate how they can exercise. This is especially important for people with limited mobility – for example, those with weakness on one side (hemiparesis) or amputations, and those using wheelchairs. The instructor pays attention to them, repeats their individual movements with other participants in the group and finally prepares the programme, which is based on these and similar (though not more difficult) movements and movement patterns. The aim is to involve all participants in the group. The whole session is accompanied by recorded music, with this initial phase requiring music that is slower and calmer.

The main part of the session is accompanied by recorded music, which is, alternately, faster and slower, according to the needs of all participants. The instructor suggests some movements to the rhythm of the music but also welcomes other initiatives: movement, sounds, singing, clapping, laughing or anything that is spontaneously offered by all participants, including people with dementia and assistants. The intensity of dance alternates during the session according to participants' condition and concentration: some may continue 'dancing' while others may need to rest for a period or be invited to perform easier 'dance' movements.

Some elements of dance can occur whilst standing in circle, in lines or in pairs as well as when seated, where participants support each other by holding hands. Assistants are helpful here particularly when some participants choose to dance whilst standing or in pairs such as in ballroom dancing. During the session the instructor suggests gradually changing each type of exercise so that the session contains exercise fitness, balance, strength and repeated activities.

The final phase of a session is slower and it includes light exercise while sitting, and relaxation. The emphasis is on social interaction, pleasant communication and enjoying each other's company. The dance instructor concludes by thanking all participants to show appreciation for their contribution.

These basic sessional plans can be modified, but we recommend always including the three main phases – the introduction, the main dance exercises and the final relaxation. The ideal number of participants in the group is ten or fewer (depending on the number of participants who need special attention, people with dementia or people using wheelchairs). If the group is larger or if there are more people in wheelchairs or with other significant disabilities, assistance from staff, family members or volunteers is strongly recommended. The involvement of assistants is also important for the sustainability of the programme – they too have opportunity to gain from participating and engagement with others in the group.

Implementing *EXDASE*

In this section we outline our experience of implementation in a variety of settings and the obstacles that we had to overcome; consider the conditions needed for implementation in dementia care (such as qualities of the dance instructor, helpful resources and particular needs of the person with dementia); and discuss the experiences of care home staff.

EXDASE has been implemented in more than 40 facilities for older people in the Czech Republic and further afield. These include care homes, nursing homes, day units for people with dementia and hospitals. Over a third of sessions have been video-recorded and later reviewed and analysed, to ascertain participants' comfort and satisfaction, communication, adequacy of movement and safety. Although *EXDASE* was originally designed for people with a physical disability, in long-term care facilities for older people in the Czech Republic, it was quickly recognised that it could be suitable for people with dementia, since it was developed to meet the needs and abilities of all who lived in care homes, including people with severe disabilities and advanced dementia.

The rationale for adequate exercise is well known, but we found that recommendations are not generally implemented (Janečková *et al.* 2013). Reasons include 'amotivation' (known as dementia-related 'apathy'), reluctance to exercise and prejudice about its value in dementia care. The inability to attend to an activity, or to understand instructions, presents particular obstacles for people with dementia, and some may have increased activity due to agitation where they may be looking for important things, activities that they used to engage with in past times or people who may no longer be present. Here they may need different creative activities to fill their day (Rylatt 2012) (see also Chapter 6). Other factors that impede implementation are associated with changes in a person's joints and muscles, and disabilities arising from long-term illness that have restricted mobility. The instructor needs to have knowledge of all these factors and adapt approaches and related exercises for individual participants. They may also need to consider help from assistants

Successful implementation often depends on the personality and competence of the instructor, who:

- should have some knowledge of the impacts of dementia and related conditions. (Potential instructors need to be both competent and creative to deliver *EXDASE* and have a relaxed communication style to interact with people who may have difficulties with language or in sustaining attention due to dementia.)

- must be able to select and compile music for the whole programme

- should have a sense of humour and the ability to communicate, both verbally and particularly non-verbally, and express a sense of belonging, politeness, respect and partnerships (between instructor and participants, assistants and others)

- must be able to react to challenges, notice feelings and appreciate humorous and entertaining ideas.

When exercising with participants from different cultures, the instructor needs knowledge of these cultures and should respect these.

For example the instructor may need to alter ways of communicating mutual greetings and the choice of the music that is used if there are cultural or sub-cultural differences between participants. This approach is seen in the choice of dance chosen in the case study reported previously (Abreu and Hartley 2013).

So far we have described the potential for applying *EXDASE* in settings of frail people with severe disabilities and dementia. For people in the early stages of dementia, the programme is similar to that for older people without dementia. However, most people with dementia appear to enjoy and succeed though immediate imitation of movement, rather than when longer movement variations are used. Thus avoiding long tasks and movement sequences and dancing together with the instructor or an assistant can be helpful.

Although the optimal group size for delivering *EXDASE* is small (six to eight people with advanced dementia or those that are wheelchair users, eight to ten with mild dementia or with other disabilities), in reality this can depend on the context of the care setting. Indeed, the programme may be useful in much larger groups of sometimes up to 30 participants if there is involvement of assistants such as staff, volunteers or family members.

Case Study 13.1 – **Mr Miroslav**[1]

Mr Miroslav has been living in the care home for six years. He has many health problems, including painful symptoms arising from his diabetes, trouble with his eyes and problems with his sight and hand movement following a stroke. After his stroke, he was not able to continue his much loved hobby of woodcarving – at which he was very accomplished. He became depressed and subsequently a 'problem' for care workers who were not able to cope with his mood and depression (despite antidepressants).

When dance classes were introduced in the care home, he initially refused to take part. Later he became curious and started to participate. Then he found that the impaired mobility of his right hand or his impaired vision did not matter hugely in dancing. He was listening to music that reminded him of his student days. He loved to dance then. And now – he could dance. The dance instructor understood his active

---

1   Names in case studies in this chapter are pseudonyms.

nature and invited him to help him support others in a circle, then to invite ladies to dance and then... Mr Miroslav regained his interest in life. He became very involved in preparing the sessions and persuading other residents to dance. His mobility and coordination improved and generally he felt much better.

Positive experiences can be seen for staff and those observing (see Projekt GOS 2010). As sessions progressed, we observed better communication between all participants and improved mood, sometimes moments of joy, expressed verbally or non-verbally through facial expressions or gestures. *EXDASE* appears to be acceptable to people engaged with it and some were willing to participate where they declined traditional exercise programmes and physiotherapy.

Our experience of *EXDASE* and its emotional effect showed some unexpected positive results where non-verbal, and sometimes verbal communication and reminiscing in people with dementia had occurred. These have been pleasantly surprising for care staff as the following comments illustrate:

'Often we discover a previously unknown ability of our clients. Let us tell of one episode from our department. The dance instructor turned on the CD player and started to prepare a dance programme. Before she had started to communicate with the participants, Mr W rose and invited her to dance. He danced two dances and everybody was very surprised, because Mr W suffered from advanced dementia and almost no other activities had been attractive to him. He did not usually get involved, he mostly slept, almost never communicated verbally and walked very poorly. It was for all of us a really big surprise.' (Care home worker, Strážnice)

'The more trust they feel the more important and interesting they are. Unfortunately, some of their peers see it as "showing off", but we can always remove this doubt. The dances are prepared so that everybody can master them. We dance with both wheelchair users and walkers. It is beautiful and they are all great and wonderful.' (Care worker in an older people's care centre, Hodonin)

'For staff, it is a big surprise to find out how introverted clients and clients with communication problems can suddenly have fun in the group.' (Manager of a care home for older people, Božice)

The contribution of the dance programme is perceived as extremely positive. Older people and professionals alike are interested in *EXDASE* and actively participate:

'Exercise through dancing confirmed to us the idea that if we provide older people with dementia with the right conditions and if we give them enough confidence, the results often enhance skills and abilities, and give a sense of their dignity and social importance, which in care facilities, they are often more or less deprived of.' (Manager of a care home for older people, Černá Hora)

Prevention of adverse effects

We initially approached delivery of *EXDASE* very cautiously. Our team geriatrician was aware of potential adverse effects and offered guidance such as the correct positioning of limbs and wheelchairs to avoid tipping the head backwards, and recommendations about the need to gradually rise during position changes. This guidance was used in structuring the exercise sessions. Attention was also paid to safe and adequate footwear, the environment where the exercise takes place, the removal or absence of barriers, and the quality of mobility aids. We suggest that if the instructor and assistants adhere to these basic measures, adverse effects are unlikely to occur.

We have not had serious adverse effects such as sudden health complications or falls during the programmes, which have involved more than 1500 older people in different care settings. Invitations to dance have mostly been accepted without potential protestations such as 'I hate dancing, I hate music'. However, *EXDASE* is a voluntary activity and the refusal to participate is not considered an adverse event. Sometimes a person with dementia leaves the session, especially if the group is too large to offer them individual attention – this should be noted and addressed if possible.

Despite few adverse effects on participants, similar to other studies (Guzmán-García *et al.* 2013) we too found some negative staff attitudes. Often it was possible to prevent these attitudinal obstacles, such as where the home managers had decided to run the sessions and the care workers were aware that they were going to take place. However, problems can arise and are difficult to overcome. This is seen in Case Study 13.2, which also illustrates the value of preparing staff to help bring them on board, and also the way in which such efforts can be sabotaged.

Case Study 13.2 – Jana

Jana, an experienced and skilled dance instructor, carefully prepared the dance session for the new care home which she was about to visit. She received some preliminary information about the home's residents. She prepared music and some tools (simple 'music instruments'). She introduced herself to the Director at the home and the care workers. Despite the positive attitudes of the Director and some care workers, the senior care worker's attitude was clearly negative. She repeatedly explained that for 'their residents' a dance session was not convenient. She was not helpful in communication with staff and even discouraged them. Despite all Jana's efforts, after five dance sessions with declining numbers of participants, and despite the fact that those present enjoyed dancing, it was agreed not to continue in this effort. The Director apologised but did not address the cause, which in Jana's view was the negative attitude of the senior care worker.

Conclusions

The programme proved a useful component of care for people with dementia in different types of care provision. *EXDASE* may not only provide helpful movement and fitness but may also improve mood and enhance enjoyment. The programme should be individualised according to the abilities and needs of the participants. An ongoing three-arm randomised controlled trial is taking place in Hong Kong to compare dance versus exercise versus no intervention in people with dementia (Ho *et al.* 2015). Future trials could evaluate the effects of *EXDASE* with people with dementia, their family, friends and care providers on outcomes such as movement, psychosocial health and falls.

Acknowledgements

The research project on quality of care and dignity in long-term care institutions is supported by the grant NT11325 of the Ministry of Health of the Czech Republic and by the Charles University in Prague research support projects P20 and P38.

References

Abreu, M. and Hartley, G. (2013) 'The effects of Salsa dance on balance, gait, and fall risk in a sedentary patient with Alzheimer's dementia, multiple comorbidities, and recurrent falls.' *Journal of Geriatric Physical Therapy 36*, 2, 100–108.

Cameron, I., Gillespie, L., Robertson, M., Murray, G. *et al.* (2012) 'Interventions for preventing falls in older people in care facilities and hospitals.' *Cochrane Database Systematic Reviews 12*, 12, CD005465.

Coaten, R. (2001) 'Exploring reminiscence through dance and movement.' *Journal of Dementia Care 9*, 19–22.

Coaten, R. and Newman-Bluestein, D. (2013) 'Embodiment and dementia – dance movement psychotherapists respond.' *Dementia 12*, 6, 677–681.

Christofoletti, G., Oliani, M.M., Gobbi, S., Stella, F., Bucken-Gobbi, L.T. and Renato Canineu, P. (2008) 'A controlled clinical trial on the effects of motor intervention on balance and cognition in institutionalized elderly patients with dementia.' *Clinical Rehabilitation 22*, 618–626.

DiLauro, M., Pereira, A., Carr, J., Chui, M. and Wesson, M. (2017) 'Spousal caregivers and persons with dementia: Increasing participation in shared leisure activities among hospital-based dementia support program participants.' *Dementia 16*, 1, 9–28.

Duignan, D., Hedley, L. and Milverton, R. (2009) 'Exploring dance as a therapy for symptoms and social interaction in a dementia care unit.' *Nursing Times 105*, 30, 19–22.

Dupuis, S.L., Whyte, C., Carson, J., Genoe, R., Meshino, L. and Sadler, L. (2012) 'Just dance with me: An authentic partnership approach to understanding leisure in the dementia context.' *World Leisure Journal 54*, 3, 240–254.

Gillespie, L.D., Robertson, M.C., Gillespie, W.J., Sherrington, C. *et al.* (2012) 'Interventions for preventing falls in older people living in the community.' *Cochrane Database Systematic Reviews 12*, 9, CD007146.

Guzmán-Garcia, A., Hughes, J. C., James, I. A. and Rochester, L. (2013) 'Dancing as a psychosocial intervention in care homes: A systematic review of the literature.' *International Journal of Geriatric Psychiatry 28*, 9, 914–924.

Guzmán, A., Freeston, M., Rochester, L., Hughes, J.C. and James, I.A. (2016) 'Psychomotor Dance Therapy Intervention (DANCIN) for people with dementia in care homes: A multiple-baseline single-case study.' *International Psychogeriatrics 28*, 10, 1695–1715.

Guzmán-Garcia, A., Mukaetova-Ladinska, E. and James, I. (2013) 'Introducing a Latin ballroom dance class to people with dementia living in care homes, benefits and concerns: A pilot study.' *Dementia 12*, 5, 523–535.

Hamill, M., Smith, L. and Röhricht, F. (2011) 'Dancing down memory lane: Circle dancing as a psychotherapeutic intervention in dementia – a pilot study.' *Dementia 11*, 6, 709–724.

Hernandez, S.S., Coelho, F.G., Gobbi, S. and Stella, F. (2010) 'Effects of physical activity on cognitive functions, balance and risk of falls in elderly patients with Alzheimer's dementia.' *Revista Brasileira de Fisioterapia 14*, 1, 68–74.

Ho, R.T., Cheung. J.K., Chan, W.C., Cheung, I.K. and Lam, L.C. (2015) 'A 3-arm randomized controlled trial on the effects of dance movement intervention and exercises on elderly with early dementia.' *BMC Geriatrics 15*, 1, 127–133.

Hokkanen, L., Rantala, L., Remes, A.M., Harkonen, B., Viramo, P. and Winblad, I. (2008) 'Dance and movement therapeutic methods in management of dementia: A randomized, controlled study.' *Journal of the American Geriatric Society 56*, 4, 771–772.

Holmerová, I., Machacova, K., Vaňková, H., Veleta, P. *et al.* (2010) 'Effect of the Exercise Dance for Seniors (EXDASE) program on lower-body functioning among institutionalized older adults.' *Journal of Aging and Health 22*, 1, 106–119.

Janečková, H., Dragomirecká, E., Holmerová, I. and Vaňková, H. (2013) 'The attitudes of older adults living in institutions and their caregivers to ageing.' *Central European Journal of Public Health 21*, 2, 63–71.

Jirák, R., Holmerová, I. and Borzová, K. (2009) *Demence a jiné poruchy paměti.* Prague: Grada.

Karkou, V. and Meekums, B. (2017) 'Dance movement therapy for dementia.' *Cochrane Database of Systematic Reviews 2*, 2, CD011022.

Machacova, K., Vaňková, H., Volicer, L., Veleta, P. and Holmerová, I. (2017) 'Dance as prevention of late life functional decline among nursing home residents.' *Journal of Applied Gerontology 36*, 12,1453–1470.

Muir, J.W., Kiel, D.P., Hannan, M., Magaziner, J. and Rubin, C.T. (2013) 'Dynamic parameters of balance which correlate to elderly persons with a history of falls.' *PLoS One 8*, 8, e70566.

O'Rourke, H., Sidani, S., Chu, C., Fox, M., McGilton, K. and Collins, J. (2017) 'Pilot of a tailored dance intervention to support function in people with cognitive impairment residing in long-term care: A brief report.' *Gerontology & Geriatric Medicine 3*, 1–8.

Palo-Bengtsson, L. and Ekman, S.L. (2002) 'Emotional response to social dancing and walks in persons with dementia.' *American Journal of Alzheimer's Disease and Other Dementias 17*, 3, 149–153.

Projekt GOS (2010) Terapeutický tanec se seniory, lektor pan Veleta úterý. Accessed on 15/6/2018 at www.youtube.com/watch?v=m7KnQncU6ik

Ravelin, T., Isola, A. and Kylmä, J. (2013) 'Dance performance as a method of intervention as experienced by older persons with dementia.' *International Journal of Older People Nursing 8*, 10–18.

Rosler, A., Seifritz, E., Krauchi, K., Spoerl, D. *et al.* (2002) 'Skill learning in patients with moderate Alzheimer's disease: A prospective pilot-study of waltz-lessons.' *International Journal of Geriatric Psychiatry 17*, 12, 1155–1156.

Rylatt, P. (2012) 'The benefits of creative therapy for people with dementia.' *Nursing Standard 26*, 33, 42–47.

Stephan, I. and Amthor, L. (2011) 'Dancing while sitting: Quality of life and health training – singing, swinging, swaying.' *Pflege Z, 64*, 6, 338–340.

Suchá, J. and Holmerová, I. (2016) 'Psychomotorická terapie u seniorů s demencí.' *Physical Culture/Telesna Kultura 39*, 1.

Vaňková, H., Holmerová, I., Andel, R., Veleta, P. and Janečková, H. (2008) 'Functional status and depressive symptoms among older adults from residential care facilities in the Czech Republic.' *International Journal of Geriatric Psychiatry 23*, 5, 466–471.

Vaňková, H., Holmerová, I., Machacova, K., Volicer, L., Veleta, P. and Celko A. (2014) 'The effect of dance on depressive symptoms in nursing home residents.' *Journal of the American Medical Directors Association 15*, 8, 582–587.

Veleta, P. and Holmerová, I. (2004) *Introduction to Dance Therapy for Seniors.* Prague: Czech Alzheimer Society and Peter's Dance Centre.

Chapter 14

Psychosocial Intervention to Reduce Depression and Apathy in People with Dementia

ACT IN CASE OF DEPRESSION (AID)

Debby L. Gerritsen and Ruslan Leontjevas

Introduction

Depression and apathy are important problems in nursing homes: on average, about 29 per cent of residents have depression (Mitchell and Kakkadasam 2011), and apathy rates have been estimated at 32 to 36 per cent (Selbaek, Engedal and Bergh 2013). Overlapping but distinct (Mortby, Maercker and Forstmeier 2012), both depression and apathy are associated with adverse resident outcomes (Smalbrugge *et al.* 2006; van Reekum, Stuss and Ostrander 2005). Thus, identifying and treating depression and apathy in residents are necessary but they often go unnoticed in nursing and care home settings. Staff may have other priorities, or they may not consider the residents' depression or apathy as 'a problem', or they may attribute the symptoms to dementia, or to other illnesses, or to functional impairments (AGS/AAGP 2003; Thakur and Blazer 2008).

For depression, collaborative care and additional psychotherapy are more beneficial than pharmacotherapy (medication) alone (Oestergaard and Moldrup 2011). Nevertheless, most nursing home residents with depression are treated solely with antidepressants (Levin *et al.* 2007). This is a striking finding, since there is little evidence for the effectiveness of antidepressants among nursing home residents (Boyce *et al.* 2011) and for people with dementia (Banerjee *et al.* 2011). In contrast, there is growing evidence that psychosocial strategies are effective for depression and apathy in residents with and without dementia living in long-term care facilities (e.g. Bharucha *et al.* 2006; Brodaty and Burns 2012), and that such strategies have minimal side-effects. Therefore, the treatment of depression and apathy for nursing home residents should include non-pharmacological approaches.

With depression as a starting point, the multidisciplinary care programme 'Act in case of Depression' (AiD) was developed by Nijmegen University's long-term care network (UKON). UKON is collaboration between 15 care organisations and the Department of Primary and Community Care of the Radboud University Medical Centre in The Netherlands (Gerritsen *et al.* 2011). Since there have been positive effects of AiD on apathy (Leontjevas *et al.* 2013b), the programme now also incorporates apathy care. AiD contains procedures about how to detect depression and apathy, pathways for psychosocial and pharmacological treatment strategies, and a procedure for monitoring the effects of a given treatment.

This chapter describes AiD, summarises its acceptability, feasibility and evaluation and considers implementation, including sustainability and delivery in other countries.

Act in case of Depression (AiD): A care programme for the detection and treatment of depression and apathy

The primary goal of AiD is to reduce depression, and it has also been shown to reduce apathy and increase residents' quality of life. The management of depression and apathy is improved by improving expertise in nursing-home practitioners and by providing a set of rules to coordinate how the different disciplines should work together in assessment and in providing treatment. AiD has three pillars. First, the programme is evidence and practice based: it is an applicable elaboration of current national and international guidelines (AGS/AAGP 2003) and scientific evidence. Since nursing home staff had extensive input in developing the programme, it has a good fit with routine daily practice. Second, the programme is tailored to the individual resident, taking into account their cognitive status and specific needs. Third, AiD is a multidisciplinary programme. It is essentially a rational decision-making approach (see Chapter 2) for procedures that different practitioners (e.g. nursing and care staff, activity therapists, psychologists and physicians) can use in a coordinated approach to the management of depression and apathy in care homes.

We will describe AiD and the learning from a large cluster-randomised trial in The Netherlands (the AiD trial: see Gerritsen *et al.* 2011; Leontjevas *et al.* 2013a). An important aspect of AiD is that it provides a set of rules with an algorithm for actions but leaves room in each step for clinical expertise in deciding whether to proceed to a next step (see also Chapter 2 on rational decision-making for selecting individualised psychosocial intervention and care planning for people with living at home). Furthermore, assessment scales and treatment protocols are suggested, but can be replaced by new or adapted instruments and protocols if these have been shown to be valid and effective.

Assessment procedures

AiD assessment has three elements. The first two elements constitute a two-step screen to recognise or detect residents with probable depression or depressive symptoms, or apathy. The third element is an extensive diagnostic procedure for those residents who have been recognised as probably depressed or apathetic during screening.

The first assessment step, 'Detection', is performed by nurses twice a year. AiD advises the use of an observer-rated instrument that primarily focuses on non-verbal symptoms. This is because residents with dementia may have substantial communication impairments, particularly in expressing their feelings, and because the use of self-reported scales can be impractical in routine practice and everyday care. In the AiD-trial, the Nijmegen Observer Rated Depression Scale (NORD) was used because it is sensitive, short and easy to score (Gerritsen *et al.* 2012) The NORD can be used on a regular basis among residents with and without dementia. Recently, a question on apathy was added to the NORD, in order to start assessment of apathy within the AiD-cycle.

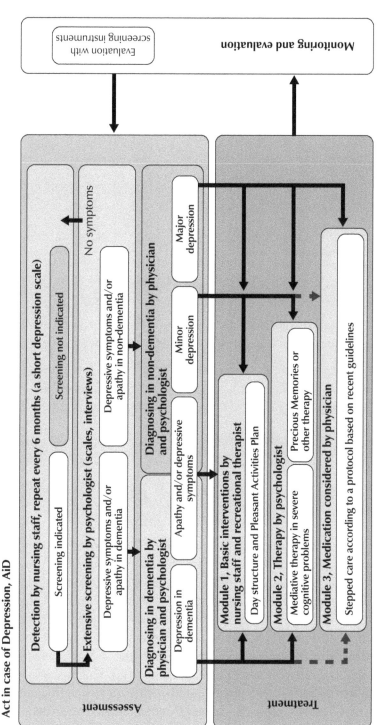

Figure 14.1: A rational decision-making procedure for AiD (Leontjevas et al. 2013a).

The Nijmegen Observer Rated Depression (NORD) Scale (Leontjevas *et al.* 2012c)

Instruction: Answer 'yes' when the behaviour was present in the last two weeks, and 'no' when the behaviour was not present or not applicable to your client. 'Often' means that the behaviour was present for several hours during at least eight days of the last two weeks.

1. Does the client often look sad, gloomy or cheerless?

2. Does the client often cry or is he/she often emotionally distressed?

3. Does the client often lack a positive response to social contacts or pleasant events?

4. Does the client often need to be encouraged to do something or participate in joint activities?

5. Does the client often have problems with sleep (falling asleep, maintaining sleep, waking up) or appetite (no appetite, unusually hungry)?

If more than one question is answered with 'yes', further screening is indicated.

6. Are there other signs to suspect depression?

7. Are there signs of apathy?

If the answer to questions 6 and/or 7 is 'yes', further screening is indicated.

The second assessment step, 'Screening', should be conducted by a psychologist when this is indicated by the previous step. Also, if a professional still suspects a depression but the detection instrument indicates otherwise, this second step can be conducted. AiD advises the use of self-report screening instruments if the severity or type of cognitive or other impairments allow for this, alternatively a proxy-based instrument is advised. During the AiD-trial, the interview-based Geriatric Depression Scale eight-item version (GDS8: Jongenelis *et al.* 2007) was used for those who could be interviewed, with a cut-off score of >2; and the Cornell Scale for Depression in Dementia (CSDD:

Alexopoulos *et al.* 1988), for those who could not be interviewed, with a cut-off score of >7. Because the CSDD has been validated in people with and without dementia, its use is not restricted to people with dementia. Additionally, the shortened version of the Apathy Evaluation Scale with 10 items (AES-10: Lueken *et al.* 2007; Marin, Biedrzycki and Firinciogullari 1991) was used and validated in residents of both dementia and non-dementia care units. A cut-off score of >21 indicated apathy among residents of non-dementia units and >29 among residents with dementia (Leontjevas *et al.* 2012a).

The third element of AiD assessment is a diagnostic procedure undertaken by a psychologist and a physician. This starts with the screening instruments in 'Screening' or when the two professionals decide to start the procedure based on additional information provided by the nursing home staff, the resident or another source. Because depressive symptoms in people with dementia can be different from those in people without dementia, the Provisional Diagnostic Criteria for Depression in Alzheimer's Disease were used in the AiD trial for residents with dementia (Olin *et al.* 2002), while the Diagnostic and Statistical Manual of Mental Disorders was used for residents without dementia (APA 2000). For apathy, the Proposed Diagnostic Criteria for Apathy in Alzheimer's Disease were suggested (Robert *et al.* 2009).

Treatment strategies

For treatment, AiD prescribes a multidisciplinary approach (see Figure 14.1) and emphasises psychosocial treatment. Treatment is evaluated in multidisciplinary meetings between physicians, psychologists and nursing and care staff in the home. The AiD algorithm includes three treatment modules for depression. The first is also applicable for apathy; in the AiD trial that module appeared effective for apathy.

- *Module 1*: Environmental and behavioural strategies by nursing or care staff and/or an activity therapist, to be started for residents with depressive symptoms or depression, or apathy.

- *Module 2*: Treatment by a psychologist. Module 2 is complementary to Module 1 for residents who meet the criteria for a depression diagnosis (minor depression, major depression, or depression in dementia).

- *Module 3*: Consideration of pharmacological treatment by a
  doctor. This is complementary to Modules 1 and 2 for residents
  with major depression or very severe depressive symptoms, or
  when psychosocial treatment Modules 1 and 2 are not effective
  enough. AiD emphasises the need for psychosocial treatment
  prior to pharmacological treatment.

For Module 1 (environmental and behavioural strategies), AiD provides
guidelines for and examples of a Pleasant Activities Plan (PAP) and a
Day Structure Programme (DSP). Those can be used by the care staff
(Teri *et al.* 1997; Verkaik *et al.* 2009). A DSP aims at structuring daily
activities and avoiding disruptions in circadian (day and night) rhythm.
The PAP aims to involve the resident in activities that they consider
pleasant and avoid activities they consider unpleasant. Nursing home
staff set initial goals (such as 'the client socialises with other residents')
and they explore and describe how these can be attained. In this
process, information about the resident from personal files and from
interviews with the resident and significant others, such as family
members, should be used.

In Module 2, if communication with the resident is possible, therapy
starts with an individual session between a resident and a psychologist.
In this session, the psychologist explores whether 'talk therapy' is
applicable. It should be noted that it is *not* a diagnosis of dementia that
determines the chosen treatment, but the resident's communicative and
cognitive abilities. If possible, the psychologist initiates talk therapy.
In the AiD-trial, Precious Memories therapy (Bohlmeijer *et al.* 2010)
was recommended, a form of life review therapy adapted for nursing-
home residents. It is based on the concept that retrieving, reaffirming
and validating positive memories in the context of present-day life may
help treat depression. A depressed person may have over-generalised
negative autobiographical memories, and training to retrieve specific
positive memories may improve their mood (see Haber 2006 for a
theoretical discussion of this). For residents with severe communicative
and cognitive problems, a 'mediation' approach may be the only option.
In 'mediation therapy', the psychologist treats a client by changing
(mediating) their (social) environment. In nursing homes, this can
be done by educating and advising nursing and care staff. Through
analysing the resident's behaviour, the professionals can develop tools
or information about ways to re-interpret and cope with depressive

behaviour, and to react in a way that benefits both the resident and the staff. The mediation therapy protocol of AiD follows Hamer's framework (2003).

The third treatment module of AiD suggests consideration of the use of antidepressants, complementary to Modules 1 and 2, but only if the resident's depression is very severe, especially in residents with dementia. National and international evidence-based pharmacological guidelines should be used. The Dutch AiD pharmacotherapy protocol stresses caution in prescribing antidepressants for residents with dementia; there is no strong evidence that antidepressants are effective in this group (Banerjee *et al.* 2011). Treatment effects need to be evaluated after four weeks. Furthermore, a psychiatrist should be consulted in cases of psychotic symptoms, suicide attempts or food refusal. This is also the case if prescribed medication remains ineffective and/or when a lithium addition is considered.

Evaluation and monitoring

The third component of AiD is the multidisciplinary evaluation of treatment and monitoring. Evaluation is done at a time point set by the psychologist and physician when treatment is initiated. For the evaluation of treatment results, AiD proposes the use of the assessment instruments and diagnostic criteria applied in the assessment procedures. Furthermore, in addition to nursing home staff being alert for depressive symptoms and apathy, monitoring also helps staff observe the treatment's feasibility and results.

Case Study 14.1 – **Mrs Berg**[1]

Mrs Berg is a 78-year-old woman living in the dementia unit of a nursing home, diagnosed with Alzheimer's disease. Although she was well loved and very much engaged in daily life of the unit, the staff noticed that she was getting more agitated during morning care, was awake during several hours in the night and was drowsy during the day and wanted to remain in her room. A nurse decided to fill in the NORD. The score of 3 indicated further assessment by a psychologist. After AiD assessment procedures, depression in Alzheimer's disease was diagnosed.

---

1   This case study has been anonymised.

The staff informed and educated her family about the condition, adapted her day programme's structure, and made a Pleasant Activities Plan with a focus on social contacts and daylight, being outdoors and physical exercise. A psychologist talked to Mrs Berg, in which it became clear that talk therapy would not be possible, but that social contacts were very important for her. The psychologist started mediative therapy with the care team. After analysing the behaviour of Mrs Berg and the care team, two goals were formulated: the first was to involve her more in her own Activities of Daily Living, especially during morning care; the second was to involve her in daily chores and helping other residents. In successive sessions with the psychologist, the staff learned together how to provide Mrs Berg's morning care by encouraging her independence as much as possible.

On evaluation of this treatment, it appeared that her circadian (changes in day and night) rhythm had been restored and her depressive symptoms decreased. Staff continued using the Pleasant Activities Plan and Day Structure Programme. Mrs Berg did not require antidepressants.

The AiD-trial

Between May 2009 and March 2011, the effects of AiD were tested in a multicentre, stepped-wedge cluster-randomised trial, which was conducted in 17 dementia special care units and 16 units for physically frail residents (somatic units) in nursing homes in The Netherlands. The primary endpoint was depression prevalence, which was determined by the proportion of residents per unit with a score of more than 7 on the Cornell Scale for Depression in Dementia. Secondary outcomes were depressive symptoms (also measured by the Cornell), health-related quality of life (Visual Analogue Scale (VAS) of the Euroqol-5D outcome measure), and apathy (Apathy Evaluation Scale-10 items) (Leontjevas et al. 2012a).

Outcome

An effect-size of 0.2 (the difference between group means – i.e. average, divided by the pooled standard deviation at baseline) can be interpreted as the minimum clinically important difference one tends to find between a new treatment and an alternative standard treatment

(Kazdin and Bass 1989). The AiD-trial showed effect-sizes larger than 0.2 for depression outcomes, quality of life and apathy. In nursing home units for frail older people (somatic units) the AiD programme reduced depression prevalence (using the statistical test of effect size, Cohen's d, –0.6), along with the severity of depressive symptoms. Also, residents' self-reported quality of life improved due to the programme (Cohen's d, 0.4) in both dementia special care and somatic units. Noticeably, a higher implementation rate of depression assessment procedures was associated with larger effect sizes (Cohen's d, –1.1 for depression prevalence in somatic units). Further, in dementia units, the AiD programme reduced apathy (Cohen's d, –0.4). There was an indication that psychosocial interventions (Module 1 and 2) can be used effectively in reducing depression and apathy in both somatic and dementia units. However, this was not found for the pharmacological treatment module. Moreover, there was an indication that pharmacological treatment may even worsen apathy. These results highlight the necessity of multicomponent and multidisciplinary care programmes and prudence in using antidepressants.

Implementation

For implementation, three types of strategies were used in the AiD trial:

1. *Information*: The research team delivered printed and digital material tailored for the stakeholders: psychologists, physicians, and nursing home staff, including the unit manager and activity therapists.

2. *Education*: The nursing home staff attended a three-and-a-half-hour training course about depressive symptoms and AiD. In this course, specific attention was paid to recognition of depression, using observational scales and supporting residents with depressive symptoms or depression through applying treatment Module 1. A training course on Precious Memory Therapy was offered to the psychologists. A medication protocol was presented to the unit physician, who was contacted by phone to discuss the protocol with a physician involved in the protocol development.

3. *Tailored communication*: In 'content interviews', physicians and psychologists were invited to discuss possible questions about the

programme content. Unit managers were contacted by phone to remind their staff to start a new assessment cycle ('Detection'). In feedback interviews, individual scores on depression screening scales and the progress of the treatment modules were discussed with the psychologists.

Relevance and feasibility

A process evaluation of the AiD-trial showed that stakeholders were satisfied with the programme (Leontjevas *et al.* 2012b). Most of the stakeholders would recommend the programme as it stands or some of its individual elements to other colleagues. Nursing home staff and the other main stakeholders (physicians, psychologists and unit managers) all reported that depression awareness and knowledge about depression improved among staff. A psychologist commented: 'Awareness of depressive symptoms has increased in nursing staff…and the same holds for openness to discuss depression.'

The relevance and feasibility reported by the stakeholders imply that AiD has good external validity. However, the need for additional time to implement the programme was a barrier according to two out of five stakeholders. This is not surprising as 'insufficient time on the job to implement new ideas' is one of the most frequently named missing items in nursing-intervention research (Kajermo *et al.* 2010)

Drawbacks to implementation

Although important effects of AiD were found, and the programme was evaluated as relevant and feasible by unit managers, physicians and psychologists (Leontjevas *et al.* 2012b), implementation in nursing homes was suboptimal. In total, depression assessment was undertaken almost twice as often (76% of the indicated cases) as treatment modules (40%). Thus, treatment was not started in more than half of the indicated cases. Module 2 was provided in somatic (non-dementia) units (49%) almost three times as often as in dementia units (17%); a Day Structure Programme and a Pleasant Activities Plan were developed and conducted more often in dementia units (48%) than in somatic units (35%) (Leontjevas *et al.* 2012b). The stakeholders mentioned several reasons for suboptimal implementation: high workload and limited time; collaboration problems between the disciplines; frequent staff changes; unfulfilled positions for psychologists and/or physicians; non-constructive role of management; reorganisations; team instability; and variable attitudes towards the programme.

In the AiD trial, the implementation approach was heavily reliant on the intrinsic motivation of health professionals and included education, feedback and reminders, and tailored communication for the professionals involved. Our stakeholder interviews suggest that additional and different implementation approaches are needed to increase extrinsic motivation and to ensure that the homes' managers provide the time needed by their staff.

The AiD programme: Recommendations for implementation

We identified three elements that should guide the implementation process of a multicomponent, multidisciplinary intervention such as AiD:

- adequate allocation of roles

- feasible arrangements

- timely evaluation.

Allocation of roles

Implementing an innovation in nursing homes requires the involvement of several stakeholders. First, a project leader is needed to coordinate the implementation. This project leader may be a local opinion leader or may be helped by one. Second, nursing home managers must be involved, not only in approving the implementation, but also in facilitating it. For nursing home managers, supporting a stable multidisciplinary staff group and empowering them are crucial factors when introducing care-improvement programmes. Investment in educational strategies and in activities for residents is necessary. Third, regarding innovative care programmes and AiD specifically, staff education is needed. This, as well as the work of nursing staff in the implementation process of AID, needs to be facilitated by the managers. Fourth, psychologists and physicians must take the lead in carrying out programme elements and make sure treatment is being evaluated. A final crucial stakeholder is the resident and their relatives, to whom the implementation strategies should be tailored, enabling them to be involved in providing treatment, for instance in facilitating and carrying out the Pleasant Activities Plan (Verkaik *et al.* 2011).

Feasible arrangements

It is important to make a specific time schedule for implementation of the programme, which includes training of those involved and providing them with information. Given the barriers we found in the AiD trial, a local analysis prior to the implementation is very important. This can provide insight into the expectations of all stakeholders, their way of communication and cooperation, and can identify possible barriers to changing working routines. After this, agreements must be made that are written down and incorporated into the nursing home's current guidelines and regulations.

Evaluation

Lack of evaluation is a major barrier to providing care of high quality in general and implementing care innovations in particular. Often, treatment strategies in nursing homes are not evaluated, resulting in problems persisting and being under-treated. A solid working routine in which evaluation meetings are structurally planned may improve evaluation and timely adjustment of treatment. Evaluation of the implementation process itself is crucial when implementing a new way of working: this must be evaluated at several time points during the implementation. To optimise implementation, it might be useful to start with implementing a programme in one nursing home unit and, after a given period of time, to evaluate whether and how it can be spread out into the whole organisation.

Application of AiD in other countries

AiD outlines pathways for procedures and offers suggestions for their content. The suggested screening instruments and treatment protocols may not be valid in countries other than The Netherlands. Thus, before implementing AiD in other countries, it is necessary to critically reflect on the AiD protocols using national guidelines and expertise.

A potential drawback for implementation in other countries may be that long-term care in The Netherlands is highly multidisciplinary, with psychologists and elderly care physicians being employed by, and present in, the care organisations. In other countries, a unit manager may have an important coordinating role in implementing AiD, including requesting assistance from psychologists and/or physicians.

Conclusions

To date, only a few complex intervention studies have been attempted in a nursing home setting – a setting with high rates of staff turnover, reorganisation and low investment in staff education. The current economic challenges may delay the improvement of depression and apathy care because squeezed budgets can result in limited staff time and staff vacancies. Nevertheless, it is not always a matter of needing major additional resources when improving care. For instance, the first screening step using a short observer-based screening instrument takes only a few minutes of staff time for each resident, and the routine use of AiD will require less time as staff expertise grows. In our opinion, it is important to think in terms of what we can actually do, which is: Act in case of Depression.

Acknowledgements

Parts of this chapter have been previously published in:

Gerritsen, D.L., Leontjevas, R., Zwijsen, S.A., Koopmans, R.T.C.M. and Smalbrugge, M. (2017) 'Depression in Nursing Home Residents with Dementia.' In S. Schüssler and C. Lohrmann (eds) *Dementia in Nursing Homes* (Chapter 13, pp.179–189). Basel, Switzerland: Springer International.

Leontjevas, R. (2012) *Act in Case of Depression! Validation and Effectiveness of a Multidisciplinary Depression Care Program in Nursing Homes.* PhD thesis. Nijmegen: Radboud University.

Leontjevas, R., Gerritsen, D.L., Smalbrugge, M., Teerenstra, S., Vernooij-Dassen, M.J.F.J. and Koopmans, R.T.C M. (2013) 'A structural multidisciplinary approach to depression management in nursing-home residents: A multicentre, stepped-wedge cluster-randomised trial.' *Lancet 381*, 9885, 2255–2264.

References

AGS/AAGP (2003) 'The American Geriatrics Society and American Association for Geriatric Psychiatry recommendations for policies in support of quality mental health care in U.S. nursing homes.' *Journal of American Geriatrics Society 51*, 1299–1304.

Alexopoulos, G.S., Abrams, R.C., Young, R.C. and Shamoian, C.A. (1988) 'Cornell Scale for Depression in Dementia.' *Biology and Psychiatry 23*, 3, 271–284.

APA (2000) *Diagnostic and Statistical Manual of Mental Disorders* (4th edn, Text Revision.) Washington, DC: American Psychiatric Association.

Banerjee, S., Hellier, J., Dewey, M., Romeo, R. *et al.* (2011) 'Study of the use of anti-depressants for depression in dementia: The HTA-SADD Trial – a multicenter randomised double-blind placebo-controlled trial of the clinical effectiveness of sertraline and mirtazapine.' *Lancet 378*, 403–411.

Bharucha, A.J., Dew, M.A., Miller, M.D., Borson, S. and Reynolds, C. (2006) 'Psychotherapy in long-term care: A review.' *Journal of the American Medical Directors' Association 7*, 9, 568–580.

Bohlmeijer, E., Steunenberg, B., Leontjevas, R., Mahler, M., Daniël, R. and Gerritsen, D. (2010) *Dierbare Herinneringen: Protocol voor Individuele life-review therpaie gebaseerd op autobiografische oefening.* Enschede: Universiteit Twente.

Boyce, R.D., Hanlon, J.T., Karp, J.F., Kloke, J., Saleh, A. and Handler, S.M. (2011) 'A review of the effectiveness of antidepressant medications for depressed nursing home residents.' *Journal of the American Medical Directors' Association 13*, 4, 326–331.

Brodaty, H. and Burns, K. (2012) 'Nonpharmacological management of apathy in dementia: A systematic review.' *American Journal of Geriatric Psychiatry 20*, 549–564.

Gerritsen, D.L., Smalbrugge, M., Teerenstra, S., Leontjevas, R. *et al.* (2011) 'Act in case of Depression: The evaluation of a care program to improve the detection and treatment of depression in nursing homes.' Study Protocol. *BMC Psychiatry 11*, 1, 91.

Haber, D. (2006) 'Life review: Implementation, theory, research, and therapy.' *International Journal of Aging and Human Development 63*, 19, 153–171.

Hamer, T. (2003) 'Mediathietherapie. De beste stuurlui staan aan wal.' In B. Miesen, M. Allewijn, C. Hertogh, F. de Groot and M.R van Wetten (eds) *Leidraad Psychogeriatrie* Part B/C (pp.414-437). Houten: Bohn Stafleu Van Loghum.

Jongenelis, K., Gerritsen, D.L., Pot, A.M., Beekman, A.T. *et al.* (2007) 'Construction and validation of a patient- and user-friendly nursing home version of the Geriatric Depression Scale.' *International Journal of Geriatric Psychiatry 22*, 9, 837–842.

Kajermo, K.N., Bostrom, A.M., Thompson, D.S., Hutchinson, A.M., Estabrooks, C.A. and Wallin, L. (2010) 'The BARRIERS scale – the barriers to research utilization scale: A systematic review.' *Implementation Science 5*, 32.

Kazdin, A.E. and Bass, D. (1989) 'Power to detect differences between alternative treatments in comparative psychotherapy outcome research.' *Journal of Consulting Clinical Psychology 57*, 1, 138–147.

Leontjevas, R., Evers-Stephan, A., Smalbrugge, M., Pot, A.M. *et al.* (2012a) 'A comparative validation of the abbreviated Apathy Evaluation Scale (AES-10) with the Neuropsychiatric Inventory apathy subscale against diagnostic criteria of apathy.' *Journal of the American Medical Directors' Association 13*, 3, 308, e301–e306.

Leontjevas, R., Gerritsen, D.L., Koopmans, R.T., Smalbrugge, M. and Vernooij-Dassen, M.J. (2012b) 'Process evaluation to explore internal and external validity of the "Act in case of Depression" care program in nursing homes.' *Journal of the American Medical Directors' Association 13*, 5, 481–488.

Leontjevas, R., Gerritsen, D.L., Vernooij-Dassen, M.J., Teerenstra, S., Smalbrugge, M. and Koopmans, R.T. (2012c) 'Nijmegen Observer-Rated Depression Scale for detection of depression in nursing home residents.' *International Journal of Geriatric Psychiatry 27*, 10, 1036–1044.

Leontjevas, R., Gerritsen, D.L., Smalbrugge, M., Teerenstra, S., Vernooij-Dassen, M.J.F.J. and Koopmans, R.T.C M. (2013a) 'A structural multidisciplinary approach to depression management in nursing-home residents: A multicentre, stepped-wedge cluster-randomised trial.' *Lancet 381*, 9885, 2255–2264.

Leontjevas, R., Teerenstra, S., Smalbrugge, M., Vernooij-Dassen, M.J F.J. (2013b) 'More insight into the concept of apathy: A multidisciplinary depression management program has different effects on depressive symptoms and apathy in nursing homes.' *International Psychogeriatrics 25*, 12, 1941–1952.

Levin, C.A., Wei, W., Akincigil, A., Lucas, J.A., Bilder, S. and Crystal, S. (2007) 'Prevalence and treatment of diagnosed depression among elderly nursing home residents in Ohio.' *Journal of the American Medical Directors' Association 8*, 9, 585–594.

Lueken, U., Seidl, U., Volker, L., Schweiger, E., Kruse, A. and Schroder, J. (2007) 'Development of a short version of the Apathy Evaluation Scale specifically adapted for demented nursing home residents.' *American Journal of Geriatric Psychiatry 15*, 5, 376–385.

Marin, R.S., Biedrzycki, R.C. and Firinciogullari, S. (1991) 'Reliability and validity of the Apathy Evaluation Scale.' *Psychiatry Research 38*, 2, 143–162.

Mitchell, A.J. and Kakkadasam, V. (2011) 'Ability of nurses to identify depression in primary care, secondary care and nursing homes: A meta-analysis of routine clinical accuracy.' *International Journal of Nursing Studies 48*, 3, 359–368.

Mortby, M.E., Maercker, A. and Forstmeier, S. (2012) 'Apathy: A separate syndrome from depression in dementia? A critical review.' *Aging Clinical and Experimental Research 24*, 305–316.

Oestergaard, S. and Moldrup, C. (2011) 'Improving outcomes for patients with depression by enhancing antidepressant therapy with non-pharmacological interventions: A systematic review of reviews.' *Public Health 125*, 6, 357–367.

Olin, J.T., Schneider, L.S., Katz, I.R., Meyers, B.S. *et al.* (2002) 'Provisional diagnostic criteria for depression of Alzheimer disease.' *American Journal of Geriatric Psychiatry 10*, 2, 125–128.

Robert, P., Onyike C.U., Leentjens, A.F.G., Dujardin, K. *et al.* (2009) 'Proposed diagnostic criteria for apathy in Alzheimer's disease and other neuropsychiatric disorders.' *European Psychiatry 24*, 98–104.

Selbaek, G., Engedal, K. and Bergh, S. (2013) 'The prevalence and course of neuropsychiatric symptoms in nursing home patients with dementia: A systematic review.' *Journal of the American Medical Directors' Association 14*, 161–169.

Smalbrugge, M., Pot, A.M., Jongenelis, L., Gundy, C.M., Beekman, A.T. and Eefsting, J.A. (2006) 'The impact of depression and anxiety on well being, disability and use of health care services in nursing home patients.' *International Journal of Geriatric Psychiatry 21*, 4, 325–332.

Teri, L., Logsdon, R.G., Uomoto, J. and McCurry, S.M. (1997) 'Behavioral treatment of depression in dementia patients: A controlled clinical trial.' *Journals of Gerontology B 52*, 4, 159–166.

Thakur, M. and Blazer, D.G. (2008) 'Depression in long-term care.' *Journal of the American Medical Directors' Association 9*, 2, 82–87.

van Reekum, R., Stuss, D.T. and Ostrander, L. (2005) 'Apathy: Why care?' *Journal of Neuropsychiatry and Clinical Neurosciences 17*, 7–19.

Verkaik, R., Francke, A.L., van Meijel, B., Ribbe, M.W. and Bensing, J.M. (2009) 'Comorbid depression in dementia on psychogeriatric nursing home wards: Which symptoms are prominent?' *American Journal of Geriatric Psychiatry 17*, 7, 565–573.

Verkaik, R., Francke, A.L., van Meijel, B., Spreeuwenberg, P.M., Ribbe, M.W. and Bensing, J.M. (2011) 'The effects of a nursing guideline on depression in psychogeriatric nursing home residents with dementia.' *International Journal of Geriatric Psychiatry 26*, 7, 723–732.

Chapter 15

Improving the Physical Environment of Care Homes

THE EVAL'ZHEIMER MODEL OF INTERVENTION DESIGN GUIDELINES

Kevin Charras

Introduction

Attention to the role of the physical environment in dementia care has led to a conceptual update of the broad arena of psychosocial interventions, with a discussion paper on eco-psychosocial interventions (Zeisel *et al.* 2016). The Eval'zheimer model of intervention has its roots in the combination of environmental psychology with clinical gerontology. The general assumption underlying this model of intervention relies on the belief that the wellbeing of people with dementia living in care homes or hospitals greatly depends on fulfilment of their daily needs as defined by Kitwood (1997), where physiological, psychological and neurological conditions are considered alongside the social, physical and organisational support provided by care facilities (Calkins 2001; Zeisel and Raia 2000).

Before considering complex and costly interventions to treat psychological and/or behavioural disorders it is important to provide a way to respond to basic needs that could contribute to these (Charras *et al.* 2010). Algase and colleagues outline a 'need-driven behavioural model' (Algase *et al.* 1996), where *need-driven behaviours* in dementia include wandering, vocalising and physical aggression. They suggest that 'unmet needs' occur when *proximal factors* in the personal, physical and social environment are incongruent with *background factors* such as neurological, cognitive, general health and psychosocial conditions.

In line with this approach, some of the disabilities experienced by people with dementia could be associated with deficiencies of the social and physical environment (Elmstahl, Annerstedt and Ahlund 1997; Passini *et al.* 2000). Designing humane and enabling physical care environments for people with dementia to meet in part some of their everyday needs, could be one step towards contributing to the complexity of providing good psychosocial, sensory and medical care for people with dementia living in care homes.

This chapter will first outline the challenges of providing environmental adaptations to meet the everyday needs of people with dementia. The second part will present an overview of theoretical and empirical aspects of designing enabling environments to provide support for people with dementia and those caring for them in institutional settings. Finally, we describe how the Eval'zheimer model of intervention combined caring practices with environmental design.

Addressing the daily needs of people with dementia

Meeting our daily needs can be quite simple, although to do so may require complex organisational, cognitive, behavioural and motor skills. They often connect to activities of daily living, such as bathing, dressing, cooking, doing chores around the house, relating with others, and so on. These needs are fulfilled by daily routines and constitute significant indicators of security, health, wealth and social status. Klumb and Maier (2007) suggest that daily activities are consistent markers of mental and physical decline as well as survival in old age. These authors maintain that household chores involving others to receive social recognition may be a marker of survival. Hence, daily activities contribute to one's survival in much the same way that, for example, not eating or unhealthy eating (see also Chapter 17), living in dirty conditions and/or social withdrawal may jeopardise general health, with the potential to contribute to physical and psychological conditions such as malnutrition, depression, cognitive decline, bacterial infections and bone fracture. Supporting this suggestion, Boumendjel and colleagues in their study *In Frigo Veritas* (*truth in the fridge*) note that the contents and state of the refrigerators of older people living at home are strong predictors of the frequency of hospitalisation (Boumendjel *et al.* 2000; Onnée *et al.* 2009).

Although Hippocrates said 'nutrition will be your primary medicine', as is also suggested in Chapter 17, this can also apply to other primary needs that form part of daily living activities. Achieving daily living activities (ADLs), however tedious they might seem, also relates to one's perception of being capable of meeting one's own needs. Not being able to achieve ADLs due to a physiological or psychological condition is a strong signal of decreasing ability to address one's basic needs for survival. Gitlin and colleagues used the *life span theory of control* (Heckhausen and Schultz 1995) in a home intervention, to demonstrate that preserving activities of daily living and instrumental activities of daily living (ADL/IADL), as well as securing the home environment, significantly increases the life expectancy of people with cognitive disorders (Gitlin *et al.* 2006; Gitlin *et al.* 2009). These authors explain their findings in two ways: first, by securing the home environment the risks of domestic accidents are reduced, although this alone cannot explain higher survival rates; second, giving a sense of control over daily life through ADLs/ IADLs could enable people with cognitive disorders to recognise their abilities to take care of themselves, thus reinforcing homeostatic mechanisms related to survival (Gitlin *et al.* 2006; Gitlin *et al.* 2009).

Much earlier, Langer and Rodin (1976) showed similar results for alertness, wellbeing and motivation in 'institutionalised' elders who were encouraged to take decisions about their daily care, compared with others who were not or those who were mostly cared for by staff. The authors point to 'iatrogenic-induced' harm resulting from healthcare provision or institutions through the malignant psychological and physiological factors and mechanisms of *learned helplessness* in people with dementia. Learned helplessness is not irreversible and can be improved by providing social and physical environments that encourage people to take part in significant activities and take some control over their lives. Thus, *occupational* opportunities provided by the environment and *comfort*, such as a sense of control, confidence and physical comfort required to engage in occupation, are important in maintaining wellbeing in people with dementia living in care facilities.

Kitwood (1997) noted that meeting subjective needs such as attachment, integration and identity also ensures a good quality of life. This can occur daily through ADLs/IADLs (i.e. being useful to oneself and others), social interactions with staff, family, friends and peers, or through the sense of security provided by shelter or personalisation of the environment according to socio-cultural norms and values. Shelter for people with dementia is found in care facilities such as special care units, retirement homes and nursing homes, where many live out their lives.

Taking a common domestic perspective, the 'home' represents the central landmark from which inhabitants plan and organise their movements from one place to another. Home is a place in which we can express and experience extended and full control, privacy, rest, security and identity. Most institutional settings for people with dementia are unfortunately unable to provide both aesthetically and practically what a home environment can offer. The reasons for this are multiple and cannot be attributed simply to care providers consciously not wishing to provide an agreeable environment. Causes of dementia-*unfriendly* environments are multidimensional due to: lack of knowledge of people–environment relationships and how to meet the environmental needs of people; restrictive security and hygiene standards; demanding families who may hold misleading beliefs about what their relative needs; budgetary restrictions; and constraining organisational and institutional policies that prioritise professional needs and safety over resident needs and safety.

Designing supportive environments
Programming enabling environmental design

Theories from environmental psychology suggest that the underlying relationships between humans and their environment are a complex system comprising social, spatial and temporal dimensions. Our social and physical environment needs to fit with our needs. Most people without cognitive disorders are able to moderate their environment according to their daily needs and aspirations. This ability requires complex cognitive abilities (identification, planning) to identify needs, causes of the needs and potential solutions available in the environment to respond to identified needs.

In order to adapt our environment, we have to be familiar with it and able to exercise enough control over it to perceive that there are opportunities to change it. Combining neuropsychological health and the living conditions of people with dementia in care homes and hospitals can drastically challenge abilities to adapt living environments according to one's needs. All conditions are brought together, organisational issues and security and hygiene standards can get in the way. Thus, a holistic environmental approach is important to embrace all of the conditions necessary to enhance wellbeing (Calkins 2001).

Understanding use of space

From the design perspective, environments are planned in order to fit their users' assumed needs. Architects and architectural programme managers need to pay particular attention to the meaning of words used to describe their needs in order to fit the main contractor's requirements. Environmental design of facilities for people with dementia could be thought about as being on a binary continuum comprising working conditions versus living conditions (Figure 15.1) where architectural programmes could be planned as working spaces in which people live, or living spaces in which people work. Depending on where in the working–living space continuum we stand at, the designed environment has to fit the differing needs. At the *working* end of the continuum, organisational issues commonly arise; whereas on the *living* end, human issues are valued.

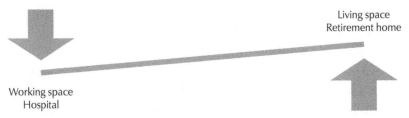

Living space
Retirement home

Working space
Hospital

Figure 15.1: Working–living space continuum of environmental design

When linking care practices to such an approach, each end of this continuum may also be seen as emphasising the semantic difference between 'taking care of' as a technical skill and 'caring for' as a humanistic attitude (Charras and Gzil 2013). Thus, we can assume that in the case of most facilities for people with dementia, words that are used to describe needs are actually often related to those of professionals (illness, care, nursing, medicine, organisation, administration) than to the daily needs of residents (comfort, identity, integration, attachment, occupation).

Professionals working in the field of dementia care often seek 'recipes' for designing dementia-friendly environments. Marshall (1998) and Fleming and Purandare (2010), demonstrate that by adopting an approach that refers to ergonomics or prosthetics, some design characteristics may complement the strengths and abilities of people with dementia by minimising and/or compensating for the effects of their neurological changes. In everyday life we also encounter and cope with the constraints of our environments according to our cultural, social and societal values. This is also the case for people with dementia. Thus, even if an environment is ergonomically adapted to a person's deficiencies, it might not correspond to their perceived needs. Additionally, what meets one person's needs might not meet those of another, and facilities for people with dementia are not aimed at solely one person but at a group of people.

This question of group versus individual needs gives rise to many debates worldwide. Some experts think 12 residents is the optimal number for a care facility, arguing that this enables people to get to know each other and helps with organising activities; others propose up to 30 residents, arguing that this enables more stimulation and favours a sense of community; while others suggest that seven or fewer is the optimal number to achieve restful and secure environments that have a home-like or family-like feeling. Although economics and the profit-earning capacity of a facility undeniably influence such choices, this debate is also one of strong cultural and individual values. Whereas collectivism is acceptable in some cultures and for some people, individualism is favoured in others, and this can be observed in the tolerance that people with dementia may express towards density in what is perceived as an *over-crowded* (excessive abundance of people compared to the availability of space), *under-crowded* (excessive abundance of space, compared to the number of users), or *equilibrated* environments (Barker 1968).

Barker (1968) suggests that the use of space is significantly determined by cultural standpoints and what might appear acceptable in one culture might not be in another. The concept of *use of space* takes its roots in archaeology and implicitly refers to Barker's (1968) *theory of behaviour settings*. To investigate habits of ancient civilisations, archaeologists have analysed the structure of the habitat in order to deduce the behavioural schemes that might have taken place in them (Rapoport 1990). Barker (1968) observed that individual behaviour is better explained by the environment in which it occurs than by investigation of individual characteristics alone. People are an essential component of the structure of a designed space and arrange their settings according to their malleability and constraints. Use of space can thus be characterised by the way an individual or a group of individuals invest and model a space according to the activities they wish to perform in it and their aspirations (Charras *et al.* 2011). Thus, *quality of use* refers to the congruency between a built space and its occupants. As argued by Barker (1968), settings are vectors of psychological, behavioural and social pressure for their users in the sense they enable and/or constrain a range of acceptable social and behavioural schemes.

Lawton and Nahemow's (1973) ecological model of ageing illustrated this pressure when they observed that adapted behaviour is the result of the interrelations of individual abilities with 'environmental press'. In other words, the fit or congruency between individual ability to process a task and the ability to cope with the inherent pressure of the environment in which the task is processed (designated as the 'adaptation level') is predictive of potential performance as well as of the emotional consequences resulting from it. This model is widely used by environmental psychologists and occupational therapists. It throws up an interesting framework to analyse the adaptive value of an environment toward its users and to make changes to enhance quality of use.

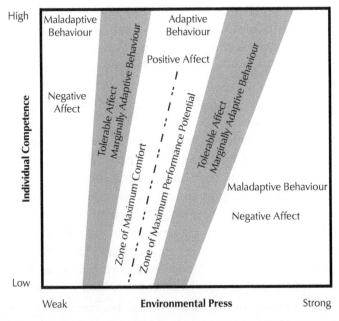

Figure 15.2: Ecological model of ageing (Lawton and Nahemow 1973)

Use of space consequences of neurocognitive and sensory alterations

Altered brain areas and cognitive processes, as well as sensory deficits, together and independently, may also have dramatic consequences on human–environment relationships. For example, cerebral areas related to exploration of the surrounding environment (rhinal and peri-rhinal cortex) (Ranganath *et al.* 2004) can change early in the course of dementia. These areas, by facilitating recognition and identification of environmental stimuli, make it possible to filter familiar information about the environment in order to focus on relevant cues that the individual might need for behavioural and cognitive processing in a given environment.

Neurological damage due to dementia can also have negative effects on environmental information processing and so affect the way people with dementia use their environment. Planning daily living activities (making a cup of tea or coffee, using the microwave, going to an appointment, and so on), for example, requires complex cognitive processing mainly based on environmental information and human–environment interrelations.

Sensory perception can also change in old age and be affected by altered sensory information processing in dementia. Poor contrasts between elements of the designed environment, confusing noises coming from multiple sources, poor lighting, and so on, can be very challenging for someone who has difficulties processing the information coming from their environment. This may lead to unexpected outcomes in the way the person uses the space they are in.

Thus, when these alterations occur, 'legibility' of the environment becomes an important factor in helping individuals to process information coming from it and to adapt behaviours according to the required behaviours that are prompted by a given setting and to use the environment in an adapted way. Building a legible environment requires understanding the standards of the person with dementia in order for it to feed back relevant cues to its users. In addition to legibility, a *prosthetic approach* can help promote safety, comfort and autonomy by maintaining the functional levels of people with dementia by taking account of their neurological, cognitive and sensory deficits (Guaita and Jones 2011).

Sometimes understanding of neurological, cognitive and sensory deficiencies can result in manipulation of the space being used by people with dementia to make life easier for care providers. Examples include darkening or bringing in light at corridor ends to encourage people to invest in some places more than others (generally for professional ease of care), painting black patches at the bottom of the doors that can be perceived as gaps to stop people trying to open them, designing 'wandering loops', building a fake bus stop for people to sit down and wait for the bus or painting *trompe-l'oeil* furniture to prevent people with dementia spoiling furniture. These 'innovations' are not without their critics who see this in terms of Kitwood's 'malignant social psychology' (1997) with questions about the ethics of taking advantage of a person's deficiencies to orient the way they use the space in their own home.

The Eval'zheimer model of intervention design guidelines

Eval'zheimer is a psychosocial model of intervention developed by the Fondation Médéric Alzheimer in France. It adapts care practices and environmental design for people with dementia living in care facilities. This model is based on the general assumption that non-pharmacological factors, such as interior design and care practices, can help reduce the behavioural and psychological symptoms of dementia. The model not only adopts a person-centred care and personhood approach but also encourages care staff to consider people with dementia as their older 'alter-egos' that need to be supported more intensely throughout daily life. To do so, environmental design is a powerful tool that supports such practices by changing the behaviour of all its users including residents, staff and families.

This idea is simple and, as mentioned earlier in this chapter, the assumption relies on the fact that we behave in different ways according to whom we sense the setting belongs to, as well as behavioural schemes and procedural knowledge that are attached to the structure of the setting (Barker 1968; Fiske and Linville 1980). The sense of control that results from ownership automatically regulates the range of behaviours each person adopts, with respect to other people (Moser 2009). If residents have the feeling that they are the owners (or shared owners) of the environment, their sense of control will enable them to exercise their rights over it. If others have the sense that the environment they are using belongs to residents, they will try and refer to the owners' norms in order to adapt their own behaviour. Legibility of the setting will equally activate behaviour schemes and procedural knowledge related to each place: for example, we do not behave in the same way and use the space in an intimate setting such as a bedroom or bathroom, as we would in a social and shared setting such as the dining or sitting-room.

On the basis of this assumption, the Eval'zheimer model of intervention design guidelines comprises six environmental dimensions based on use of space to analyse and model settings for people with dementia living in care facilities (Table 15.1). Each of the primary dimensions is then subdivided into secondary dimensions. Dimensions of the model of intervention refer to the physical and social environment to ensure congruency between expressed needs of the users (residents, staff and families) and the environmental support provided. According to their positions on the working–living space continuum, environmental design responses for each dimension will differ.

Table 15.1: Environmental design guidelines of
the Eval'zheimer model of intervention

Primary dimensions	Secondary dimensions
Structure of space Structure of space relates to physical and symbolic division of space enabling its users to represent themselves and to use the place in which they evolve, according to their norms and values and with socially adapted means.	Quantity and variability of spaces: Ratio between the number of common spaces and their diversity in terms of use.
	Accessibility of spaces: The way the space/design enables and facilitates independent access to different places by residents (gardens, living spaces, kitchen, corridor, moving spaces).
Space-induced social cohesion Social cohesion through space relates to the congruence between structure of spaces and uses that are made of it to facilitate social relationships, adapted behaviours and care of residents.	Shared spaces: Degree to which spaces are shared and facilitate social relationships between residents, as well as between care workers and residents.
	Congruency/legibility: Facilitation and support through legibility of space of adapted behaviours of residents and professionals within their social relationships and caring relationships.

cont.

Primary dimensions	Secondary dimensions
Atmosphere Domestic or institutional atmosphere can be characterised by the physical and social features of the setting.	Usage: Investment and modelling of a setting by residents and care workers according to the activities they wish to do in it and the status they are attributed and that they attribute to themselves.
	Appearance: Relates to the way the furniture, the layout and the material feed back to the perceived atmosphere.
Privacy Privacy relates to the quality of a setting as it is experienced, perceived and embraced by its occupants according to their intimate and personal characteristics.	Intimacy: Relates to possibilities of withdrawal and of regulation of social relationships enabled by the setting (opening/closure of the setting, distance from the living rooms and from the rest of the group and/or community).
	Appropriation of space: Degree to which space enables residents to establish their landmarks, to express their identity and their status toward the group and/or the community.
Display of care The way care is displayed within a setting enables to observe the balance of the relationships between care workers and residents (assistance, authority, collaboration, empathy) in its physical and social dimensions.	Professional positioning: Physical and social position of care workers toward residents and furniture used to support this position (e.g. standing behind a resident during an activity to control their behaviour, positioning objects or furniture in the sight of residents in such a way that they can or cannot use them).
	Vocabulary: Type of vocabulary used by professionals (natural/familiar, technical/professional) in the presence of residents.
Control–Attention Control implies supervision and surveillance of residents within their own spaces to keep them secure as well as to optimise institutional functioning. Attention can be defined as an attitude supported by the physical, social or organisational environment, through which professionals are encouraged to direct their attention toward residents and oversee successful relationships with others and their environment.	Common spaces: The interior design can more or less enable supervision of the global activity of the place.
	Private spaces: The way the use of the space and/or the attitudes of care workers encourage or not – or even forbid –access to these spaces by the residents.
	Professional spaces: The way these spaces are used, or can be used, for overseeing, supervision and surveillance of residents or not.

Although therapeutic outcomes from such guidelines can probably be observed, their primary aims are to ensure comfort and wellbeing to enhance quality of life of people with dementia living in care facilities (Charras *et al.* 2011). The design guidelines of the Eval'zheimer model of intervention refer to Dumur, Bernard and Boy's (2004) dimensions of comfort:

- *equipment comfort*, linked to satisfaction of primary needs

- *aesthetic comfort*, which is subjective and depends on individual perceptions

- *social comfort*, which corresponds to the balance between being with others and intimacy

- *conformity comfort*, which identifies social belonging to a group.

As emphasised by the second and the fourth dimension of comfort, the fact that these guidelines are not culture-specific makes it possible to apply them according to norms and values underlying the culture in which they are implemented. Whilst security, hygiene, fire and sanitary regulations exist, these guidelines can be used to tailor regulations and design to account for the resident's personal and cultural needs.

Conclusions: The environmental approach to dementia

Approaching dementia care through an environmental perspective demonstrates the important relationship between the person with dementia and their environment, in the same way as this occurs for everyone else. Neurological changes caused by dementia simply call for environments that are particularly easy to understand in order to compensate for cognitive, behavioural and sensory deficits. Such a statement questions the specificity of such settings inversely to its generic value. When designing facilities for people with dementia, contractors, architects and architectural programme managers should also be aware of the impact of the setting on other people's behaviour (staff, families) that can in turn impact on caring relationships. Finally, the evaluation of design characteristics of caring facilities for people with dementia should take in account the way the environment is experienced by its users and how these facilities enable daily routines to take place in order to preserve a sense of control, efficacy and contribution to others.

References

Algase, D., Beck, C., Kolanowski, A., Whall, A. *et al.* (1996) 'Need-driven dementia-compromised behavior: An alternative view of disruptive behavior.' *American Journal of Alzheimer's Disease 11*, 6, 10–19.

Barker, R.G. (1968) *Ecological Psychology: Concepts and Methods for Studying the Environment of Human Behavior.* Stanford, CA: Stanford University Press.

Boumendjel, N., Herrmann, F., Girod, V., Sieber, C. and Rapin, C.H. (2000) 'Refrigerator content and hospital admission in old people.' *Lancet 356*, 9229, 563.

Calkins, M.P. (2001) 'The physical and social environment of the person with Alzheimer's disease.' *Aging and Mental Health 5*, 1, S74–S78.

Charras, K., Eynard, C., Menez, Y., Ngatcha-Ribert, L. and Palermiti, F. (2010) 'Impact of nightshifts on quality of life of institutionalised people with Alzheimer's disease.' *Neurologie Psychiatrie Geriatrie 10*, 60, 264–269.

Charras, K., Demory, M., Eynard, C. and Viatour, G. (2011) 'Theroretical and application modalities for designing community living settings for people with dementia.' *La Revue Francophone de Gériatrie et de Gérontologie 18*, 177, 205–210.

Charras, K. and Gzil, F. (2013) 'Judging a book by its cover: Uniforms and quality of life in special care units for people with dementia.' *American Journal of Alzheimer's Disease and Other Dementias 28*, 5, 450–458.

Dumur, E., Barnard, Y. and Boy, G. (2004) 'Designing for Comfort.' In D. de Waard, K.A. Brookhuis and C.M. Weikert (eds) *Human Factors in Design* (pp.111–127). Maastricht: Shaker Publishing.

Elmstahl, S., Annerstedt, L. and Ahlund, O. (1997) 'How should a group living unit for demented elderly be designed to decrease psychiatric symptoms?' *Alzheimer Disease and Associated Disorders 11*, 1, 47–52.

Fiske, S.T. and Linville, P.W. (1980) 'What does the schema concept buy us?' *Personality and Social Psychology Bulletin 6*, 543–557.

Fleming, R. and Purandare, N. (2010) 'Long-term care for people with dementia: Environmental design guidelines.' *International Psychogeriatrics 22*, 7, 1084–1096.

Gitlin, L.N., Hauck, W.W., Winter, L., Dennis, MP. and Schulz, R. (2006) 'Effect of an in-home occupational and physical therapy intervention on reducing mortality in functionally vulnerable older people: Preliminary findings.' *Journal of the American Geriatrics Society 54*, 6, 950–955.

Gitlin, L.N., Hauck, W.W., Dennis, M.P., Winter, L., Hodgson, N. and Schinfeld, S. (2009) 'Long-term effect on mortality of a home intervention that reduces functional difficulties in older adults: Results from a randomized trial.' *Journal of the American Geriatrics Society 57*, 3, 476–481.

Guaita, A. and Jones, M. (2011) 'A "prosthetic" approach for individuals with dementia?' *JAMA 305*, 4, 402–403.

Heckhausen, J. and Schultz, R. (1995) 'A life-span theory of control.' *Psychological Review 102*, 2, 284–304.

Kitwood, T. (1997) *Dementia Reconsidered: The Person Comes First.* Buckingham: Open University Press.

Klumb, P.L. and Maier, H. (2007) 'Daily activities and survival at older ages.' *Journal of Aging and Health 19*, 4, 594–611.

Langer, E.J. and Rodin, J. (1976) 'The effects of choice and enhanced personal responsibility for the aged: A field experiment in an institutional setting.' *Journal of Personality and Social Psychology 34*, 2, 191–198.

Lawton, M.P. and Nahemow, L. (1973) 'Ecology and the Aging Process.' In C. Eisdorfer and M.P. Lawton (eds) *The Psychology of Adult Development and Aging* (6th edn) (pp.619–674). Washington, DC: American Psychological Association.

Marshall, M. (1998) 'How it helps to see dementia as a disability.' *Journal of Dementia Care* 6, 1, 15–17.

Moser, G. (2009) *Psychologie environnementale: Les relations homme–environnement.* Bruxelles: DeBoeck.

Onnée, A., Rio, C., Begel, M. and Carca, P. (2009) 'In Frigo Veritas = IN FRIGO VERITAS.' *La Revue Francophone de Gériatrie et de Gérontologie 16,* 160, 518–521.

Passini, R., Pigot, H., Rainville, C. and Tétreault, M-H. (2000) 'Way finding in a nursing home for advanced dementia of the Alzheimer's type.' *Environment and Behavior 32,* 5, 684–710.

Ranganath, C., Yonelinas, A.P., Cohen, M.X., Dy, C.J., Tom, S.M. and D'Esposito, M. (2004) 'Dissociable correlates of recollection and familiarity within the medial temporal lobes.' *Neuropsychologia 42,* 1, 2–13.

Rapoport, A. (1990) 'System of Activities and System of Settings.' In S. Kent (ed.) *Domestic Architecture and the Use of Space* (pp.9–20). Cambridge, MA: Cambridge University Press.

Zeisel, J. and Raia, P. (2000) 'Non pharmacological treatment for Alzheimer disease: A mind-brain approach.' *American Journal of Alzheimer's Disease and Other Dementias 15,* 6, 331–340.

Zeisel, J., Reisberg, B., Whitehouse, P., Woods, R. and Verheul, A. (2016) 'Ecopsychosocial interventions in cognitive decline and dementia: A new terminology and a new paradigm.' *American Journal of Alzheimer's Disease and Other Dementias 31,* 6, 502–507.

Chapter 16

Making Contact with People with Severe Dementia

MIMAKKUS – A CLOWNING INTERVENTION

Irena Draskovic and Sytse Zuidema

Introduction

This chapter outlines clowning as a person-centred non-verbal intervention for use with people in the later stages of dementia. The intervention, named 'miMakkus'[1] was piloted in nursing homes in The Netherlands. A variety of clowning techniques are used to establish interpersonal contact with people with dementia who are not able to express themselves verbally and who may also experience symptoms of agitation or depression.

Theoretical underpinnings and the programme itself are described and illustrated by two cases. Preliminary evidence is then presented with reflections on the potential for practice and research. Finally, organisational aspects for implementation are discussed, along with potential limitations of the intervention.

Theoretical underpinnings

For people with severe dementia living in nursing homes, symptoms such as agitation, depression and apathy are common, affecting about nine out of ten residents (Stewart *et al.* 2014). These symptoms present significant challenges for nursing and care staff (Chenoweth *et al.* 2009), are associated with poor quality of life for residents, and

---

1   www.mimakkus.nl

management with psychotropic drugs is of limited value due to their side-effects and other negative impacts (Ballard *et al.* 2018). In contrast, person-centred psychosocial interventions have demonstrated positive impacts on quality of life, agitation and antipsychotic use, although in advanced dementia, speech and language impairments can undermine communication and positive interpersonal contact (Brodaty *et al.* 2013). Nonetheless, the basic human needs of people with severe dementia are the same as of others: namely to feel safe, have a sense of belonging and acceptance, feel respected, and have a sense of making some kind of contribution to others (Edvardsson, Winblad and Sandman 2008). Some authors suggest that the need to 'belong' or 'belongingness', (including feelings of tenderness/affection and associated behaviour), has a distinct neural signature (Kolanovski, Fick and Buettner 2009; Kolanowski *et al.* 2011, 2012; Low *et al.* 2014). It follows then that what may help alleviate distressing symptoms is an intervention that meets the person's need to 'belong', to be accepted and to contribute in ways other than depending on their impaired cognitive 'channels'.

One factor common to successful person-centred approaches in late-stage dementia care is to reduce reliance on speech and memory as a means of communication. This requires alternative means of communication such as engaging with emotions within each interpersonal situation. This has been demonstrated in studies where if the caregiver is relaxed and smiling during intimate self-care activity, the resident remains calm and cooperative (Burgener *et al.* 1992). Also, where the caregiver allows the severely impaired resident to control the interaction, food consumption increased (Amella 1999). Behrman (2013) suggests that humour, such as that used in clowning, can have a beneficial effect on cardiovascular, respiratory and immunological responses; and on pain, memory and alertness, which boosts wellbeing and the ability to deal with stressful situations. This in turn can reduce depersonalising interactions, improve interaction with care providers, and neutralise the hierarchical 'doctor–patient' relationships that may undermine communicative efficacy in people with dementia. Thus clowning and laughter-based interventions have good potential to reduce agitation and promote happiness (Low *et al.* 2014).

Examples of successful clowning-based interventions in dementia care are emerging, such as 'The Laughter Bosses' (Brodaty *et al.* 2013), 'gericlowns' (Rösner 2010) and comedy activities (Hafford-Letchfield 2013). These kinds of approaches seem to be effective in engaging people with severe dementia in positive interactions, improving mood and alleviating dementia-related distressing symptoms (Low *et al.* 2014).

The pilot miMakkus clowning intervention stimulated more positive behavioural responses from nursing home residents with dementia than equally long friendly visits by nurses where talking predominated. The possible mechanisms underlying these effects may involve compensation for, or the fulfilment of, frustrated needs for contact (Moll *et al.* 2012). Clowning in dementia care requires little conversation, thus minimising the potential for confusing a resident whose abilities to understand and respond to verbal utterances are largely impaired. Thus non-verbal methods of communication within interactions with the person who has severe dementia and language impairments demonstrates how the person with dementia can still be reached and engaged (Edvardsson *et al.* 2008).

The miMakkus intervention

miMakkus is a Dutch clowning intervention that has been used in dementia care, motivated by the need to re-establish communication with people with impaired communication. Non-verbal techniques, such as facial expressions, sounds, songs and posture are used to help establish contact while at the same time by-passing cognitive impairments. Typical visual clown features are used sparingly in miMakkus; instead the emphasis is much more on personal contact and non-verbal communication. By doing so the risks of negative reactions are reduced. The intervention originates from an initiative in which a clowning professional tried to establish contact with residents with advanced dementia. Essentially, the assumption guiding this experiment was that genuine contact and recognition of the need for positive human contact that promotes, for example, affection, could enhance the residents', wellbeing and quality of life. On one occasion, a woman who had retained some verbal skills said: '*Hey, there'h* **my friend** *the clown again*', and thus the name miMakkus was born.

Background

In 2002, the miMakkus organisation was established and the training was developed. The focus is on learning to establish positive contact and improve wellbeing and quality of life in people with cognitive problems or functional limitations. Since 2002, over 160 trainees have been trained as miMakkus clowns. Initially, trainees were nursing home professionals, such as activity organisers, wishing to learn a new way to communicate with residents in the late stages of dementia. Gradually, those undertaking training became more diverse and training was modified into a modular approach, suitable for anyone interested in learning new forms of communication.

To become a certified miMakkus clown, following an audition, the person can enrol on a 22-day training programme, followed by a seven-day internship. However, becoming a miMakker is optional; basic communication skills can also be learned separately. Training over two to three days for family carers has also been developed. This aims to help families learn methods of non-verbal communication and to improve awareness of the impact of their interactions on the person with dementia.

miMakkers often work in nursing homes, mainly with residents who have difficulties establishing communication due to cognitive problems arising from dementia or stroke. Often in these cases family members also have difficulties in communicating with and reaching out to their relative. miMakkers have also worked with homeless people, army veterans and retired nuns.

Intervention components and basic principles

A miMakkus practitioner aspires to establish contact with people who, for different reasons, may have lost the ability or the motivation to initiate contact with others. Imagine that:

- you are dependent on others for your activities of daily living and no longer able to express your needs and wishes to those who support you

- your usual way of perceiving and interpreting the world has changed beyond recognition

- your knowledge of the world, the certainties you thought you had in life, and your sense of security are greatly reduced and you feel you are losing your very self.

What is left is a 'moment-by-moment' experience of the 'here and now'. In this new situation basic human needs for attention, warmth, understanding and shared perceptions of the world remain. What you need is a way of communicating that overcomes your cognitive limitations and people who understand this. The exact time and place are not important for meaningful communication. Instead, the opportunities to provide affectionate warm contacts with the person with dementia need to be grasped by others, including those providing care.

The principles of this intervention are to make respectful, calm, genuine emotional contact with the person with dementia. It is important to follow the person with dementia by recognising and capturing their needs and their ongoing potential for positive interaction *in situ*. A basic technique is improvisation, tuning in to the 'here and now'. Communication is mainly non-verbal, so sounds and words are often used with enhanced or different meanings. The focus is on being together, experiencing the moment together, and sharing the emotions of the moment. This type of communication usually takes the form of mime, body language, sounds and sometimes 'nonsense' words.

miMakker: Presentation and skills

miMakkers are characterised by their warm-coloured, lively looking, and not necessarily matching clothing, with make-up to accentuate their eyes and mouth. The fabric (i.e. touch and feel) of their clothes is important, since this is sometimes used to make the first contact. Other items for initiating contact include handheld puppets, musical instruments, music boxes and soft fabrics. Each miMakker uses their own set of props that reflect their personality – such as items that are 'mischievous', 'modest' or 'cheerful'. The clown's distinctive nose has a specific function; that is, to communicate the subjective realm of non-verbal emotional interaction.

Traditionally, jesters and clowns stand for primary emotions of joy or grief, for laughter and silliness, for mime and imitation, reflection and provocation. The advantage of a clown over a care worker, or even over a family member, is that its sheer appearance already sets the stage for non-standard communication. Clowns are expected to deviate from rules, social protocols and well-known standards. A clown is allowed to make mistakes: everyone laughs kindly if a clown misuses everyday objects such as using a shoe rather than a vase for holding flowers. Indeed, this subtly mirrors what can occur when a person with dementia makes a mistake; but the clown can do such things without being seen as offensive. It makes the sense of 'being different' in dementia more acceptable and perhaps easier to live with. Most of the time, people with dementia respond to clowns without difficulty. Be it smiles or even tears, the contact appears to 'touch' them and brings them and interactions into 'here and now'.

Being able to remain continuously sensitive to and tune into different residents' needs, wishes and possibilities requires concentration. To do this, a clown needs to remain 'naïve' and unprejudiced, be a keen observer of body language, properly assess a situation, and respond spontaneously and appropriately. Therefore, an important part of the training is dedicated to the skill of 'making oneself empty' and 'giving full attention to another person'.

Illustrations of miMakker in nursing homes

The following case studies outline stories of the work of clowns with people with severe dementia living in nursing homes.

Case Study 16.1 – **Mr Brown and miMakker Loeloe**[2]
'My little rascal'

Mr Brown seems to live entirely in his own world and is difficult to engage. If he is emotionally touched, this frightens him and often he reacts with agitation or even anger. He no longer takes part in activities in the home; during activities he becomes restless and usually withdraws and leaves. It seems as if he cannot enjoy anything any more. Sometimes, he flips aimlessly through the pages of a newspaper or a magazine.

Loeloe (a clown) comes into the living room and sees Mr Brown, sitting at the table, bent forward. There are newspapers on the table. It looks like Mr Brown is reading the papers, but Loeloe notices that his eyes are closed and he is asleep. Loeloe sits beside him and listens to his breathing. Today, she has a puppet dog with her. Loeloe lets the dog sniff all over the table while she provides the appropriate dog sounds. Little by little, 'the dog' comes closer to the newspapers and Mr Brown's hand. There is no reaction from him. In the meantime, the dog is sitting

---

2 Names in case studies in this chapter are pseudonyms.

on the newspapers and is making rustling noises. 'Accidentally', the dog touches Mr Brown's hand. He turns his head up and opens his eyes.

Loeloe first lets the dog face Mr Brown, then she lets it look at him from different angles and positions. Each time, Mr Brown follows the dog with his gaze. Suddenly, he lifts his hand and gently taps the dog's nose. He shakes it gently back and forth, smiles and says: 'Hello, my little rascal!' Now, he looks up and sees Loeloe and with radiant eyes he laughs. 'Did you bring Bobbie?' he asks, as Loeloe vigorously nods affirmatively. 'How good of you!' he says. He keeps on playing with Bobbie and Loeloe for quite some time.

The interaction between Mr Brown and the dog-puppet was a surprise to all. However, Mrs Brown later mentioned that they had a much loved dog called 'Bobbie'. We learned that Mr Brown used to be very fond of dogs and that the family always had a dog in the home. Having heard about the episode with the clown, Mrs Brown discovered new ways to reinstate contact with her husband using previously videoed materials of good times with the family and their dogs. The social worker organised a visit from a real dog organised by the charitable foundation Animals in Care, but Mr Brown's reaction was not entirely positive – he seemed to prefer interacting with Bobbie the dog-puppet and Loeloe or reminiscing with his wife. In addition to his beloved 'Bobbie the Dog', the essential ingredient of meaningful engagement appeared to be the way in which Loeloe interacted with Mr Brown.

Case Study 16.2 – **Miss Spring and miMakker Sophie**
'Tender without words'

Miss Spring frequently sits with her eyes closed and her head down. 'She sleeps' says her neighbour to Sophie, a miMakkus clown. When Sophie sees that Miss Spring's eyes are finally open, she sits unobtrusively next to her at the table. Slowly and quietly, Sophie slides her hand across the table and into Miss Spring's visual field. Faster than Sophie had expected, Miss Spring reacts. She lifts her right hand confidently from her lap and lays it onto Sophie's hand, and she starts to caress her gently. Sophie responds in kind, and they are both happy, tenderly stroking each other's hands; no words. Sophie invites Miss Spring's other hand to join in and this is immediately accepted. Finally, Miss Spring gently brings Sophie's hands to her mouth and kisses them lovingly. Sophie looks up and sees two most beautiful sparkling blue eyes looking back at her. It was a small gesture but of great importance to both Miss Spring and Sophie.

Reflections

Non-verbal communication with residents in end-stage dementia may help to engage them in 'real-time' social communication and reduce isolation. Low *et al.* (2014) suggest that the mechanism by which humour therapy can impact on agitation may be by addressing unmet needs for company and meaningful activity (Kolanowski and Litaker 2006). Our pilot miMakkus intervention showed that, in comparison to verbal interaction, it stimulates positive behavioural responses in people with dementia. This in itself makes it worthwhile to try to use the clowning techniques of non-verbal communication and humour in daily practice. In The Netherlands an important addition to the miMakkus intervention and its use in daily practice has been a training programme for nursing home staff. The goals of this training are to raise awareness of the specific communicative needs and potential of people with dementia; and to offer training in non-verbal communication skills. Some techniques can be incorporated into basic skills training for care staff.

Implementing clowning interventions such as miMakkus in nursing homes requires staff with positive attitudes to person-centred care. Care staff, activity organisers and nursing home managers all need to be aware of the importance of engaging people with severe dementia in meaningful activities. Managers are particularly important since they motivate others to learn new skills and can encourage a switch from task-centred to person-centred care. A basic requirement for people working with people with dementia is the recognition that besides providing care, spending time interacting meaningfully with residents or just 'being there' for them, are equally important. Clowning interventions such as miMakkus can be used if cognitive or other problems are preventing interpersonal contact and participation in social life. Clearly these should be curtailed if the person responds negatively to a clown. There may also be culture-specific responses that may need to be understood before this type of intervention can be piloted for acceptability outside The Netherlands or in people's own homes.

Acknowledgements

We thank our colleagues Annemieke van Brunschot, Caren Mannens, Myrra Vernooij-Dassen for their assistance with this chapter and study.

References

Amella, E.J. (1999) 'Factors influencing the proportion of food consumed by nursing home residents with dementia.' *Journal of the American Geriatrics Society 47*, 879–885.

Ballard, C., Corbett, A., Orrell, M., Williams, G. *et al.* (2018) 'Impact of person-centred care training and person-centred activities on quality of life, agitation and antipsychotic use in people with dementia living in nursing homes: A cluster-randomized controlled trial of the WHELD intervention.' *PLoS Med 15*, 2, e1002500.

Behrman, S. (2013) 'Have you heard the one about the man with Alzheimer's disease?' *British Medical Journal 346*, 2872.

Brodaty, H., Low, L.F., Liu, Z. and Fletcher, J. (2013) 'Successful ingredients in the SMILE Study: Resident, staff, and management factors influence the effects of humor therapy in residential aged care.' *American Journal of Geriatric Psychiatry 22*, 12, 1427–1437.

Burgener, S.C., Jirovec, M., Murrell, L. and Barton, D. (1992) 'Caregiver and environmental variables related to difficult behaviors in institutionalized, demented elderly persons.' *Journals of Gerontology B 47*, 4, 242–249.

Chenoweth, L., King, M.T., Jeon, Y.H., Brodaty, H. *et al.* (2009) 'Caring for Aged Dementia Care Resident Study (CADRES) of person-centered care, dementia-care mapping, and usual care in dementia: A cluster-randomised trial.' *Lancet Neurology 8*, 4, 317–325.

Edvardsson, D., Winblad, B. and Sandman, P.O. (2008) 'Person-centered care of people with severe Alzheimer's disease: Current status and ways forward.' *Lancet Neurology 7*, 4, 362–367.

Hafford-Letchfield, T. (2013) Funny things happen at the Grange: Introducing comedy activities in day services to older people with dementia.' *Dementia 2*, 6, 840–852.

Kolanowski, A. and Litaker, M. (2006) 'Social interaction, premorbid personality, and agitation in nursing home residents with dementia.' *Archives of Psychiatric Nursing 20*, 1, 12–20.

Kolanowski, A., Fick, D.M. and Buettner, L. (2009) 'Recreational activities to reduce behavioural symptoms in dementia.' *Geriatric Aging 12*, 1, 37–42.

Kolanowski, A., Litaker, M., Buettner, L., Moeller, J. and Costa, P.T. (2011) A randomized clinical trial of theory-based activities for the behavioral symptoms of dementia in nursing home residents.' *Journal of American Geriatrics Society 59*, 6, 1032–1041.

Kolanowski, A., Bossen, A., Hill, N., Guzman-Velez, E. and Litaker, M. (2012) 'Factors associated with sustained attention during an activity intervention in persons with dementia.' *Dementia and Geriatric Cognitive Disorders 33*, 4, 233–239.

Low, L.F., Goodenough, B., Fletcher, J., Xu, K. *et al.* (2014) 'The effects of humor therapy on nursing home residents measured using observational methods: The SMILE cluster randomized trial.' *Journal of the American Medical Directors' Association 15*, 8, 564–569.

Moll, J., Bado, P., de Oliveira-Souza, R., Bramati, I.E. *et al.* (2012) 'A neural signature of affiliative emotion in the human septohypothalamic area.' *Journal of Neurosciences 32*, 36, 12499–12505.

Rösner, M. (2010) 'The clown doctor: An introduction.' *Zeitschrift für Gerontologie und Geriatrie 43*, 1, 53–57.

Stewart, R., Hotopf, M., Dewey, M., Ballard, C. *et al.* (2014) 'Current prevalence of dementia, depression and behavioural problems in the older adult care home sector: The South East London Care Home Survey.' *Age & Ageing 43*, 4, 562–567.

Related reading

miMakkus website: http://mimakkus.nl (In Dutch)

Camp, C. and Camp, L. (2017) *Teaching Empathy and Conflict Resolution to People with Dementia: A Guide to Person-Centered Practice.* London: Jessica Kingsley Publishers.

Ellis, M., Astell, A. and Scott, S. (2019) *Adaptive Interaction and Dementia: How to Communicate Without Speech.* London: Jessica Kingsley Publishers.

James, I. and Gibbons, L. (2019) *Communication Skills for Effective Dementia Care: A Practical Guide to Communication and Interaction Training (CAIT).* London: Jessica Kingsley Publishers.

Sollberger, M., Stanley C.M., Wilson S.M., Gyurak, A. *et al.* (2009) 'Neural basis of interpersonal traits in neurodegenerative diseases.' *Neuropsychologia 47,* 13, 2812–2827.

Chapter 17

Promoting the Enjoyment
of Food in Dementia Care

THE BON APPETIT INTERVENTION IN CARE HOMES

Dana Hradcová, Michal Synek, Iva Holmerová and Jitka Zgola

Introduction

Food – its preparation, sharing and enjoyment – brings into our lives much more than just the nourishment of the body. Interpersonal relations and attention to its material dimensions are equally important in good care (Harbers, Mol and Stollmeijer 2002). Food can also play a key role in shaping cultural and social roles and is a means of creating and supporting relationships (Philpin 2011; Roberts 2011; Sader 2012). Indeed, dining with friends and family creates particular positive experiences (Curle and Keller 2010; Hung and Chaudhury 2011; Tadd *et al.* 2011).

Food is so much part of our everyday ordinary routine that important aspects other than nutrition, both in healthcare practice in general and in the care of people with dementia, can be underestimated (Walton *et al.* 2013; Watson and Green 2006). It determines the steady rhythm of the day and is a pleasurable aspect of many social situations. Shared meals are a symbol of family life and also part of important events, such as those relating to civil, religious or military ceremonies in community life. The cultural context of food can be seen in different religious practices surrounding particular foods. For example, in Christianity 'meat-free Fridays' are sometimes observed, and in other religions food practices include halal, kosher or vegan customs. Therefore food is also a way in which faith is celebrated in community life. The saying 'good food and good company' reflects the well-known enjoyable aspects of food-related social life.

People with dementia who live in care homes have the right to an ordinary personal and social life. This includes taking part in food preparation, eating where and when one chooses, choosing one's food and sharing mealtimes with neighbours, friends or where possible with family. Therefore we need to appreciate all aspects associated with food in the care of people with dementia. Adequate nutrition is, of course, an important part of health and care services; and healthy eating is an important part of a healthy lifestyle (AGE 2012). For many people with dementia, diets are prescribed, prepared and served in a hospital or a nursing or care home facility. These consumers, however, may not enjoy what is on offer (Mol 2010), or even not 'eat well' for other reasons.

Problems with eating are caused by many factors (Marshall 2003). Particular food-related challenges can occur for the person and their carer(s) throughout their journey with dementia. Of these, weight loss and difficulty in swallowing are described as the most unpleasant symptoms of dementia (Watson and Green 2006). However, the problem is not only associated with physical wellbeing, but also on how dementia influences emotional wellbeing. The ability to follow previously well-adhered-to norms of social behaviour and self-consciousness can limit opportunities for socialising. Early on, before the person with dementia exhibits significant cognitive deficits, minor problems in memory, perception and orientation may make it difficult to find the way to the dining room, to remember mealtimes, to make food choices, to maintain a socially acceptable conversation or to observe 'good table manners'. As dementia progresses, remaining seated at a table may become more difficult and it may be harder to concentrate on eating using crockery and cutlery. People with dementia often become less able to recognise the feelings of satiety or hunger, at the extreme being either oblivious to hunger or constantly craving food. Later, as a result of motor-function impairments, the person may have problems with bringing food to the mouth. Chewing and swallowing difficulties, resulting in coughing and choking are some of the most distressing problems in dementia care (Holmerová et al. 2013). These problems can contribute to a view that the target of care is simply to ensure that the person has received some nutrition.

This chapter focuses on promoting enjoyment of food by those caring for people with dementia, in long-term nursing and care home settings. It describes the Bon Appetit programme carried out in care homes in the Czech Republic. The programme did not deal solely with the nutritional aspects of food, but also on social and culturally important food values that contribute to a wider framework of care for people with dementia. The goal of well-managed care provision for people with dementia is to support the person's dignity, contact with their family and respect for their culture, always taking account of their unique and potentially changing abilities, tastes and needs (Schell and Kayser-Jones 1999) and considering how to serve food well (Manthorpe and Watson 2003). The aim of the Bon Appetit intervention (Zgola and Bordillon 2001) was to enable care home residents to receive the best possible experience from their food, including appropriate nutrition, and to offer staff the support needed in achieving these goals. The philosophy of the programme was based on the belief that 'good food' is that which is prepared by using good raw materials and served with respect to its consumers (Manthorpe and Watson 2003). Although the programme outlined was developed for use in nursing or care homes and other long-term care settings its principles can be used in hospitals where older people with dementia receive medical or mental health care.

The Bon Appetit programme

The Bon Appetit programme, striving for the enjoyment of eating whilst living in a long-term care setting, was first described by Zgola and Bourdillon (2001). The Czech translation was published by the Czech Alzheimer Society (Zgola and Bordillon 2013). This was supplemented with a chapter describing programme implementation in Czech long-term care facilities. It was implemented in the Czech Republic, in 16 long-term (care home) care settings, which typically had large numbers of residents. From the beginning, when recruiting the homes to the programme, we realised that although most people consider food an important part of life, it may not be so easy to give it the same level of importance in the lives of residents in long-term care settings. The need to pay attention to food, on the other hand, had recently been confirmed by the results of an investigation by the Office of the Public Defender of Rights (Ombudsman), carried out systematically in various areas of Czech long-term care since 2006. The risks of malnutrition and a violation of fundamental rights and dignity through inappropriate catering for people needing care were, according to the Ombudsman, a serious problem (Veřejný ochránce práv 2015).

Collaboration between various professionals and representatives from all parts of the home's workforce was a basic condition for successful implementation of the programme. However, inter-professional collaboration in long-term care was hard to establish. Therefore, the initial groups that were invited to collaborate in Bon Appetit were teams from care homes with which we had long-standing cooperation on the Dragonfly certification for quality of care (Hradcová *et al.* 2014). These facilities had been implementing assisted self-assessment in which inter-professional collaboration was a key concept.

At the beginning of the process, consultants facilitated focus groups and supported staff to carry out an assessment of current dining experiences in the care home where they worked. While it was not necessary to explain why we discussed food and dining with care workers when striving for improvements in quality of care, achieving cooks' and cleaners' involvement was not straightforward. Gradually it was understood that attention and care to 'materiality of food' and the ways food is processed, stored and delivered to consumers can enhance or diminish the pleasurable experience surrounding food. In this context, 'materiality of food' refers to what food is and does (meaning that it makes us feel happy or disgusted), to whom it is important (people who are honoured guests or prisoners) and what people do around food (whether they sit passively or make decisions or get involved in the cooking). It was important for cooks to meet with residents and to learn about their needs and preferences. Other important areas required change, such as mopping floors in a dining room when some residents were still having lunch, which was not respectful. As a result of such discoveries, the work schedule of the staff became more flexible to meet the needs of the residents. Through small changes, the vision of person-centred care was enacted, not just by means of task assignments, but through building functioning respectful relationships. The necessity for inter-professional collaboration and enhanced teamwork was appreciated by the managers, as one care home Director commented:

> 'Bon Appetit is perceived as an important piece of the mosaic of improved quality of care... I was personally surprised by the impact of the programme in other areas of care. We expected to change and increase the quality and level of catering, but we changed also many other aspects of care, where initially we did not expect any changes. The

programme in our facility linked, on a professional and personal level, different sections, staff groups and clients more than any previous effort.'

The programme implementation team in each care home consisted of representatives of care assistants and nurses, a nutritional therapist, cooks and social workers, as well as departmental heads and auxiliary and cleaning staff. Each team was asked to appoint a coordinator to facilitate the work in their care home and to communicate with the external consultants.

When implementing the Bon Appetit programme, we placed great emphasis on active involvement of all the staff of the care home and on discussing programme principles, as well as staff members' experiences and views on food and dining. At the initial stages of the programme, the project consultants visited all the 16 participating care homes and talked to the staff on several occasions about their attitudes to serving food to residents, about what food means to them personally, what they think about the residents' ability to enjoy meals, which areas of care function smoothly in their care home (in relation to food), and what they would like to change. We met with the managers at each care home as well as with frontline staff. Occasionally, refreshments were served during these meetings by the consultants. When consultants played the role of hosts and hostesses, their efforts were well received by the care home workers. Such experiences helped to facilitate an understanding of the main principle of the programme – a relational approach to care (Zgola 1999).

Later, the consultants spent time participating in and observing mealtime activities. Staff and residents became familiar with their presence, although in some homes staff continued to feel uneasy, since they perceived the consultants as 'inspectors' who would tell them 'what they had done wrong'. Consultants did not fully participate in care, since they were not trained in nursing. They played a role of a visiting friend, helping out when possible. In these situations, some staff acted as supervisors to the consultants, while others thought it was strange for the consultants to clean up or to do some of 'their work'. During feedback after a mealtime, it was very important for the consultants not to respond to requests around 'what they had done wrong and how to do it better', but rather to facilitate the exchange of ideas about 'what shall we try next?'.

Another useful activity was joint baking, which helped both the staff and the consultants to recognise the importance of practice in improving communication and relations with residents of the care homes. One consultant invited residents and care home staff to bake cakes together in the kitchen. Residents seemed to find pleasure not only from the results – delicious cherry soufflé – but also from such experiences as seeing and eating fresh cherries, or encountering fresh eggs and bags of flour on the table. These were things that they had not seen and touched for a long time, some of which had played an important part in their life before moving to the home. As one of the consultants recorded in her notes:

> 'Seemingly ungainly hands of one of the ladies grabbed an egg, cracked it over the edge of bowl and masterly separated yolk from egg white. I can remember the anxiety in the gaze of an occupational therapist, and then expression of a relief and pleasant surprise on her face, when the task was finished.'

We considered such events meaningful activities respecting the interrelationship of body with culture and history (Kontos 2006) and thus nurturing the personhood of each resident. It takes a relational approach to autonomy (Agich 2003) to do these very ordinary things well, and to enjoy them, while cherishing human dignity. Thus, based on the understanding of the care workers, who were able to recognise the importance of ordinary things in everyday life, food became our medium for further care improvements in the homes.

At the beginning of the programme, some care assistants were unable to appreciate the necessity for in-depth observations and assessment of residents' preferences and abilities, because they believed that they 'knew them very well', or they doubted the feasibility of changes related to the serving of food. The seminars and on-the-job training aimed to give the staff an opportunity to ascertain possible improvements and to assess impact of the introduced changes. As we looked closely at the practice of care and learned to value the specific features of the dining experience for each person, the programme participants – both the care workers and the consultants – realised how much tinkering (Mol, Moser and Pols 2010) was still ahead of us, if we were to take our mission seriously.

Evaluation: The quality of dining during the Bon Appetit programme

The mission formulated by its participants was 'to provide the kind of dining that enables people with dementia to eat enticing food, while respecting dignity, self-sufficiency and contact with family and other people'. The specific form of how to do this in each care home was decided by staff based on their experience and methods of monitoring care. Together they formulated a common vision, and teams from all departments and units subsequently established targets in the following areas:

- *Answering to the preferences and needs of residents and providing for their inclusion in dining*: the collation of information on favourite and disliked dishes, special needs and habits, the role of individual residents in the area of food preparation and serving, and their acknowledgement in everyday practice.

- *Food and drink*: the attractiveness, taste, texture, appearance, temperature, nutritional value, digestibility and availability of food and drink.

- *The environment*: lighting, noise, space, equipment and dining room furnishings, the layout and design of tables and chairs, table linen, crockery, and so on.

- *The social environment*: staff behaviour, resident behaviour, communication and social exchange during mealtimes, the involvement of family and friends and others.

- *Serving food*: initial welcome, methods of serving, communication, behaviour, atmosphere, special procedures and techniques for serving food, the possibility of providing specially prepared food, such as individual bites or items (finger food), pre-prepared meals, mealtime endings and cleaning.

- *Dining as individual and group restorative programme*: supplementary activities aimed at supporting socialising, stimulating the senses, specific programmes to improve the skills needed for eating food, and the ability to enjoy food.

Care home staff were asked to determine quality indicators and to create a checklist for the initial evaluation and monitoring of individual residents, of the department or work units and of the care home as a whole. With the help of these checklists, staff gradually began to see many small but important details that previously were unnoticed or overlooked. Staff needed enough time to observe carefully what happens during a mealtime in the dining room or in a resident's own room if this was where food was served. During the initial training and formulation of goals for their home, they learned how and what to observe during mealtimes and developed skills and ability to focus on important details. Each team member compiled a brief record of observations and provided feedback to colleagues. Our experience was that the skills in observation and the ability to give and receive feedback improved over time and with repetition, and that this resulted in improvements.

The responsibility for ensuring quality of care needed to be shared by everyone involved, even when communicating and receiving constructive criticism appears problematic. For many, especially the care workers, this was a new and unusual role, as they were used to receiving the feedback, not providing it. In some care homes, staff reported that working with a checklist and documentation was burdensome and unpleasant. We therefore carried out unstructured observations and, in some cases, used video as a media of analysis (e.g. Video Interaction Guidance).

Examples of observations (taken from records of Bon Appetit team meetings) that led to care improvements and increased resident satisfaction are as follows:[1]

- Some residents cannot cope with grated cheese on bread. They do not know what to do with it. They were served sliced cheese instead, while others enjoyed their bread with grated cheese.

- Diabetic jam is sometimes difficult to spread. The staff pre-mixed it, after which it became much easier to handle.

- The leaves of lettuce, even though they were cut to small pieces, fell on the table. Therefore, lettuce will be served in larger bowls.

- Mr Sladek, who is seriously ill, likes beef broth. It is offered and he is served this dish whenever he likes, day or night.

---

1   Names here and in the case study later in the chapter are pseudonyms.

- Pieces of pasta are too large. It turned out that many residents living with dementia consumed smaller-sized pieces much more easily than large pieces.

- Dining room staff were handing people sugar cubes whilst wearing a single-use plastic glove. Sugar tongs were purchased. Staff do not use plastic gloves any more while serving food in the dining room.

- An observation of serving of food on trays – *'it is impersonal, there are too many things on trays and people cannot put their arms on the table'* – resulted in agreement to serve food without trays, in a 'family style' of dining.

- Mrs Clara is now given her eye drops before her breakfast, since care assistants noticed that she was uncomfortable with itchy eyes during meals.

- Social workers and occupational therapists are now regularly seen in the dining room before and during mealtimes. They help with the preparation and serving of food, orientation, social interaction and conversation.

- A kitchenette was opened for residents on the first floor in one of the care homes. Residents can now prepare small meals for themselves, if they wish.

- Small dining rooms were arranged on each floor, so people do not have to travel all the way to the big dining hall or eat alone in their room.

Key features needed for implementation

The key preconditions for implementation of the Bon Appetit programme in the Czech context were practitioners' skills and their commitment to care about both the individuals *and* the whole experience of dining. Without courage for experimenting, patience for tinkering (Mol *et al.* 2010) and the art of holding all aspects of care in place, the joy of dining would not have been possible. Specific techniques and topics are easy to present, discuss and practise in training sessions. But it involves significant energy and motivation to continue the work in light of other possible failed efforts to deliver good care. Therefore, mutual support and acceptance of uncertainty in experimenting with new ways of food delivery were crucial.

Organisational structure of individual care homes influenced significantly the way the experience of dining was perceived and improved. The implementation teams met once every two weeks at the beginning of the programme and, later, once a month. The meetings provided opportunities to discuss input from the staff of the department or unit and to plan how to implement the changes. Once broader support for the principles of the Bon Appetit programme was reached, all staff gradually worked on identification of key values and they designed and adopted practices of good catering.

After the introductory period, the implementation teams along with consultants continued facilitation of the learning process and consulted with their colleagues, drawing on the results of observations and frontline staff recommendations. Consultants, including the author of the programme, regularly participated in various activities connected with food preparation, serving and consumption, and shared their experience with the staff members. Ongoing discussions, training and practising kept the importance of dining 'in the air' for everybody, regardless of the level of their enthusiasm.

Topics for training and consultation were determined by the members of the teams. The basic set of short training sessions included the following topics:

- food and its role in dementia care

- meals as social events

- chewing and swallowing, dealing with swallowing problems

- assessment of individual needs and planning meals for individual residents

- environment, relationships and communication at mealtimes

- assistance in dining, how to assist with helping people to eat and how to support self-sufficiency, assistive devices

- preparation of food in bite sizes, finger food, arranging food on the plate, arranging a table for residents with dementia

- food as a part of rehabilitation programmes for individuals and groups of residents

- organisation of time and workforce during mealtimes.

What worked well

In all the care homes participating in the programme, the care staff strengthened their abilities to identify and evaluate the capabilities and needs of residents. The number of people who were eating in bed decreased considerably, as did the number of people who consumed pureed food. A systematic effort can lead to substantial results, as described by one of the care home workers in Case Study 17.1.

Case Study 17.1 – **Mrs Snopkova**

Presentation of a care home worker at a Bon Appetit conference

Mrs Snopkova came to our home from the hospital. She was immobile, permanently bed-ridden, restless, anxious and sometimes aggressive, refusing care, resistive, totally dependent on care in all areas of her daily life. At mealtimes, we began to position Mrs Snopkova in bed at first, then in an armchair, and later in a chair. At the beginning of her stay the food was served to her through a syringe. Six months of care improved her ability to eat on her own, as well as her satisfaction from the food. Now Mrs Snopkova is a calm, confident woman who, with the support of staff, can meet her needs. She eats at a table where she sits with other residents.

Residents and staff appreciated the changes in the environment. 'It's beautiful; it's just like a wedding', said one resident looking at the new tables set up and nicely decorated. Residents also appreciated that in most places the staff ceased to use protective clothing and equipment when serving food (plastic disposable aprons, caps, and so on) and replaced them with colourful aprons and small caps or hats. In some dining rooms, curtains and sun-blinds were arranged to protect from direct sunlight residents who were sitting against a window. Due attention was also paid to social aspects of dining.

Residents were supported in deciding with whom and where they wanted to eat. In some care homes, they were offered several options – a large common dining room, a small dining room in the department or unit or a table in their own room to dine with a room-mate or alone. Such changes added another challenge to care workers in terms of observation and negotiations skills and flexibility. Small, family-style dining rooms were arranged in all departments or units of the care homes. As one care worker reported, 'the dining room is meant to arouse a feeling of wellbeing, it is a place where people could be happy, where they could remain seated longer to talk, to meet with others and with families'. As a result, family members attended the regular activities associated with eating (e.g. teas in the care home) more frequently, and also spent more time with their relatives.

Professionalism, autonomy and pride of care home workers was also enhanced. For example, they would independently evaluate the situation and plan the best way to assist and support residents, and they often expressed self-fulfilment and pride in their work. Cooks, who in most cases had previously spent all their time in the kitchen and had very little awareness of the tastes, preferences and needs of residents, felt more involved in care provision. They appreciated knowing for whom they were cooking, and since they now had basic information about the problems of people with dementia, they were able to understand better what they were asked to do. They began to come up with creative ways of cooking for particular residents and how to arrange the food nicely. The schedule of the care home became more flexible, more person-centred and more needs-driven.

Changes brought about by the Bon Appetit programme were summarised by a member of care staff:

'Sitting at the table with residents, sipping tea and talking, this is also our work. We have nothing to worry about when the director passes by. When we talk with residents during mealtimes, we all have a good time and they eat more, even those who do not like to eat.'

The challenges

Making a change in the general attitude to serving food and communicating with residents was the most significant challenge for care workers. Although the consultants provided a thorough explanation of the impact of dementia and repeatedly explained it in individual cases, some care workers considered it unnecessary, redundant and sometimes even embarrassing always to welcome residents into the dining room and accompany them to a table, to remind them repeatedly of, or introducing them to, whoever is sitting next to them, and to keep up a pleasant conversation whilst eating. This was particularly so for residents with severe dementia, where it seemed hard for staff to initiate or sustain friendly verbal or non-verbal interaction.

The perceived time pressures required the attention of the project team as illustrated by the following testimony, from a care staff member who found herself torn between different demands:

> 'I do not have enough time to spend with each person. Staff in the department are few, and when I have to return the dishes to the kitchen by half past one, I cannot sit with people for half an hour.'

All the facilities we worked with had over 100 residents, and some procedures and rules were firmly embedded into management cultures (for 'regimes of haste' in dining for people with learning difficulties, see Synek and Carboch 2014). In many cases, architecture and interior design in the facilities created obstacles that were hard or impossible to overcome.

Clashes between care home residents' preferences and needs and the capacity and number of staff available were sometimes inevitable:

> 'It is not that we would not like to do it better; we just do not have time to do it. I can serve the lunch to people in a dining room, but then I have to go on and serve the lunch to other residents in their room. So there is only one assistant who can help people in the dining room. All residents need at least some kind of assistance and there is just not enough of us to do it well.' (Nursing assistant, consultant's notes)

Improvements usually required organisational changes and negotiated collaboration between frontline staff and management. However, we describe examples that can appear overwhelming for staff, where the needs for care appeared to exceed the possibilities and capacities of those who are ready to respond to them. An important challenge for managers, and in our case the consultants who act as change agents, is to consider supportive regimes for residents and staff (see Beck *et al.* 2017), which may have additional benefits of minimising the negative emotional impact on staff who want to provide good care.

Conclusions

The successful implementation of the Bon Appetit programme relied on the cooperation of the entire team or work unit. Each meal, and each activity of preparing and serving food, was considered an important part of the overall care in the home and as an activity to promote dignity in people with dementia. The ability to eat is a crucial part of human life. The whole team must therefore appreciate the fact that the food should be prepared and served with respect, taking into consideration the particular capacities and needs of the person with dementia.

The Bon Appetit programme applies the principles of person-centred care to the specific areas of preparing and serving food and to related activities. Its successful implementation is based on a broad sense of caring relationships. The joy of dining requires not only taking care about people and their changing needs, but also care for taste, shape, colour and other qualities of food (Marshall 2003; Mol 2010) and how this is served (Manthorpe and Watson 2003). However, the values that the Bon Appetit programme attempted to deliver in long-term care cannot be implemented merely by applying 'golden rules of dining' or be described simply in a manual. The dining improvement programme needs to be adapted to the context of each care environment, shaped by many different human actors and physical environments. Quality of dining care in general depends on willingness to experiment continuously and to strive for 'doing better' while searching for balance between different goods, needs and possibilities. The joy of caring, the delightful emotion reminding us that we live in relationship with others (Noddings 2013), is an important aspect of this effort.

Acknowledgments

Implementation of the Bon Appetit programme was possible thanks to the support of the regional government and of the people living and working in the care homes. The research project on quality of care and dignity in long-term care institutions on which this chapter draws was supported by the grant NT11325 of the Ministry of Health of the Czech Republic and by the Charles University in Prague research support project's fund.

References

AGE (2012) *European Quality Framework for Long-Term Care Services: Principles and Guidelines for the Wellbeing and Dignity of Older People in Need of Care and Assistance.* Brussels: Age Platform.

Agich, G. (2003) *Dependence and Autonomy in Old Age: An Ethical Framework for Long Term Care*. Cambridge: Cambridge University Press.

Beck, M., Birkelund, R., Poulsen, I. and Martinsen, B. (2017) 'Supporting existential care with protected mealtimes: Patients' experiences of a mealtime intervention in a neurological ward.' *Journal of Advanced Nursing 73*, 8, 1947–1957.

Curle, L. and Keller, H. (2010) 'Resident interactions at mealtime: An exploratory study.' *European Journal of Ageing 7*, 3, 189–200.

Harbers, H., Mol, A. and Stollmeijer, A. (2002) 'Food matters: Arguments for an ethnography of daily care.' *Theory, Culture and Society 19*, 5/6, 207–226.

Holmerová, I., Baláčková, N., Baumanová, M., Hájková, L. *et al.* (2013) 'Strategie České alzheimerovské společnosti P-PA-IA.' [Strategy of the Czech Alzheimer Society P-PA-IA.] *Geriatrie a Gerontologie 2*, 3, 158–164.

Hradcová, D., Hájková, L., Mátlová, M., Vaňková, H. and Holmerová, I. (2014) 'Quality of care for people with dementia in residential care settings and the "Vážka" Quality Certification System of the Czech Alzheimer Society.' *European Geriatric Medicine 5*, 6, 430–434.

Hung, L. and Chaudhury, H. (2011) 'Exploring personhood in dining experiences of residents with dementia in long-term care facilities.' *Journal of Aging Studies 25*, 1, 1–12.

Kontos, P. (2006) 'Embodied Selfhood: An Ethnographic Exploration.' In A. Leibing and L. Cohen (eds) *Thinking About Dementia: Culture, Loss, and the Anthropology of Senility.* New Brunswick, NJ: Rutgers University Press.

Manthorpe, J. and Watson, R. (2003) 'Poorly served? Eating and dementia.' *Journal of Advanced Nursing 41*, 2, 162–169.

Marshall, M. (ed.) (2003) *Food Glorious Food: Perspectives on Food and Dementia*. London: Hawker Publications.

Mol, A. (2010) 'Care and Its Values. Good Food in the Nursing Home.' In A. Mol, I. Moser and J. Pols (eds) *Care in Practice: Tinkering in Clinics, Homes and Farms*. Bielefeld: Transcript.

Mol, A., Moser, I. and Pols, J. (eds) (2010) *Care in Practice: Tinkering in Clinics, Homes and Farms*. Bielefeld: Transcript.

Noddings, N. (2013) *Caring: A Relational Approach to Ethics and Moral Education*. Berkeley, CA: University of California Press.

Philpin, S. (2011) 'Sociocultural context of nutrition in care homes.' *Nursing Older People 23*, 4, 24–30.

Roberts, E. (2011) 'Six for lunch: A dining option for residents with dementia in a special care unit.' *Journal of Housing for the Elderly 25*, 4, 352–379.

Sader, A. (2012) *Implementing Family-style Dining*. Cleveland, OH: Institute for the Advancement of Senior Care. Accessed on 5/1/2018 at www.ltlmagazine.com/article/implementing-family-style-dining

Schell, E. and Kayser-Jones, J. (1999) 'The effect of role-taking ability on caregiver–resident mealtime interaction.' *Applied Nursing Research 12*, 1, 38–44.

Synek, M. and Carboch, R. (2014) 'Profesní slepota a režimy spěchu: Podpora soběstačnosti při jídle v institucionální péči o lidi s mentálním znevýhodněním.' [Professional blindness and regimes of haste: Support of self-sufficiency in eating in institutional care for people with mental disability.] Krompach: *Biograf, 60*. Accessed on 5/1/2018 at www.biograf.org/clanek.html?id=954

Tadd, W., Hillman, A., Calnan, S., Calnan, M., Bayer, A. and Read, S. (2011) *Dignity in Practice: An Exploration of the Care of Older Adults in Acute NHS Trusts*. Southampton: NIHR Service Delivery and Organisation Programme.

Veřejný ochránce práv [Ombudsman] (2015) *Zpráva ze systematických návštěv Veřejného ochránce práv. Domovy pro seniory a domovy se zvláštním režimem*. [Report from systematic visits in on Homes for Seniors and Homes with Special Regime.] Brno: Public Defender of Rights.

Walton, K., Williams, P., Tapsell, L., Hoyle, M. *et al.* (2013) 'Observations of mealtimes in hospital aged care rehabilitation wards.' *Appetite 67*, 16–21.

Watson, R. and Green, S.M. (2006) 'Feeding and dementia: A systematic literature review.' *Journal of Advanced Nursing 54*, 1, 84–93.

Zgola, J. (1999) *Care That Works: A Relationship Approach to Persons with Dementia.* Baltimore, MD: Johns Hopkins University Press.

Zgola, J. and Bordillon, G. (2001) *Bon Appetit! The Joy of Dining in Long-term Care.* Baltimore, MD: Health Professionals Press.

Zgola, J. and Bordillon, G. (2013) *Bon Appetit: Radost z jídla v dlouhodobé péči.* Praha: Česká alzheimerovská společnost.

Chapter 18

Awarecare

AN AWARENESS-BASED STAFF TRAINING INTERVENTION TO IMPROVE QUALITY OF LIFE FOR CARE HOME RESIDENTS WITH SEVERE DEMENTIA

Catherine Quinn and Linda Clare

Introduction

This chapter describes a staff training intervention that was designed for care home staff who work with people in the severe stages of dementia. This chapter will explore the theoretical background of the intervention and its development. It will describe the intervention and provide case examples. The final sections of this chapter will focus on the outcomes of the intervention and discuss key features needed for successful implementation.

Awareness in severe dementia

In the severe stages of dementia there are significant impairments in cognition, motor functions and verbal communication. The person is likely to be unable to clearly verbally communicate their needs and wishes and will be highly dependent on others for personal care. The later stages of dementia have sometimes been described as a 'vegetative state'; however, this does not necessary mean that people with severe dementia have reduced emotional feelings and needs (Boller *et al.* 2002). Both non-verbal communication and the ability to express emotions are often preserved to some extent in the later stages of dementia. In addition, there can be subtle signs of awareness that indicate that the person is still attending to and responding to the surrounding environment (Abramowitz 2008).

Awareness can be defined as 'a reasonable or realistic perception or appraisal of a given aspect of one's situation, functioning or performance, or of the resulting implications, which may be expressed explicitly or implicitly' (Clare *et al.* 2011, p.936). This broad definition of awareness has been operationalised in the levels of an awareness framework, with awareness operating at four levels of increasing complexity: sensory registration; performance monitoring; evaluative judgement; and meta-representation (Clare *et al.* 2011). The first of these, sensory registration, reflects the ability to register and respond to sensory and perceptual stimuli, whether relating to internal state, such as discomfort or pain, or environmental/social features, such as the presence of a familiar person or a change of temperature. It is this sensory registration level of awareness that is particularly salient for people with severe dementia who have limited or no verbal communication (Clare 2010). The demonstration of awareness at this level can be embodied in behavioural responses such as facial movements, arm movements or vocalisations, and the extent of such responsiveness is likely to be associated with dementia severity.

There is evidence that signs of awareness can be observed by both care staff and family members (Lawton, Van Haitsma and Klapper 1996). Quinn *et al.* (2013) explored how family members and care staff understand, interpret and make sense of signs of awareness in people with severe dementia. Through analysis of focus groups conducted with care home staff and family members a model of awareness emerged in which the perceived level of awareness in the person was influenced by an interaction between attributes of the person and the environment. Expressions of awareness could be hindered by environmental factors and enhanced through appropriate stimulation. Awareness was not a static state but was perceived to fluctuate, often without any pattern. Differences in interpretations of awareness were linked to the meaning assigned to particular kinds of responses. For family members, awareness was intrinsically linked to their emotional connection with the person and they would persist in seeking out signs of awareness. For care staff, identifying signs of awareness helped them to do their job and enabled them to feel that they had connected with the person.

Care staff seem to distinguish between residents whom they consider to be aware and responsive and those whom they consider to lack awareness or responsiveness (Quinn *et al.* 2013). Care staff may be less likely to try to interact with residents believed to lack awareness

(Ekman *et al.* 1991; Magai *et al.* 1996). Therefore, perceptions of awareness have potentially significant implications for resident wellbeing and quality of life (Clare 2010). One of the challenges for care staff is to feel that their interactions with people with dementia are effective and worthwhile (Hansebo and Kihlgren 2002). If care staff can be trained to identify signs of awareness in residents with very severe dementia, this should enable them to respond more effectively to the needs of the person. In addition, an appropriate level of stimulation, together with sensitive engagement by care staff, should facilitate the expression of awareness and, at the same time, enhance residents' wellbeing. Identifying signs of awareness may encourage staff to interact more with the person and may make caregiving tasks more rewarding (Clare *et al.* 2012). This may in turn enhance the quality of life of people with severe dementia.

Development of the AwareCare measure

The AwareCare intervention was developed for care home staff working with people with severe dementia. Severe dementia in this study was defined as meeting criteria for Stage 6 or 7 on the Functional Assessment Staging (FAST) (Reisberg 1988) and having no, or only very limited, verbal communication, indicated by an inability to clearly verbally communicate needs and wishes, with speech either very circumscribed and limited to single words or phrases, or completely absent.

The intervention involves care staff observing people with severe dementia using the AwareCare observational measure (Clare *et al.* 2010).[1] The AwareCare measure was developed using items from the Wessex Head Injury Matrix (WHIM: Shiel *et al.* 2000; Wilson *et al.* 2001) as a starting point. The WHIM is an observational tool originally developed to allow ward staff to monitor recovery from head injury as part of their routine clinical work by looking for evidence of clearly defined behaviours and responses. The research team examined the 62-item WHIM and identified 20 items that were the most suitable for people with severe dementia. These items were then explored in focus groups with care home staff and family members of people with dementia. An expert panel consisting of dementia care practitioners

---

1   A copy of the AwareCare observational measure can be found at http://psychology.exeter.ac.uk/reach/publications

and researchers then considered the findings from the focus groups and advised on item selection, including adaptation or substitution of items, and on formulation of the rating system. An early prototype of the AwareCare measure was piloted in the study by Clare *et al.* (2012), and from the findings of this study it was further refined.

The AwareCare measure is a matrix for recording how the person with dementia responds to environmental stimuli. It distinguishes between spontaneously occurring events (e.g. resident is spoken to) and specifically introduced stimuli (e.g. introduce one object). For each stimulus, a record is made of whether this stimulus occurred during the observation session and, if it did, the relevant responses are recorded. Responses were categorised as manifested in the eyes (e.g. makes eye contact), face (e.g. smiles), head (e.g. nods/shakes head), arm (e.g. reaches), body (e.g. moves away) or voice (e.g. mumbling). For each observation, information is also recorded about the setting in which the observation occurred and any additional behavioural responses, not covered in the matrix, that were observed.

The AwareCare intervention

The AwareCare intervention was conducted in a cluster-randomised trial (Clare *et al.* 2013) involving eight privately owned care homes in North Wales. Four of these care homes were randomised to receive the AwareCare intervention. The intervention took place over an eight-week period. In weeks 1 and 2, care staff participated in two 90-minute training sessions led by an accredited trainer. In these sessions, staff were encouraged to consider the nature of residents' awareness, were introduced to, and instructed in the use of, the AwareCare observational measure, and were given guidance on developing their skills in communicating with severely impaired residents. Staff practised using the measure between the two sessions by observing residents in the care home. In session 2, staff members reflected on any difficulties they encountered whilst conducting their practice observations. Staff members were each given an individualised schedule for observing during weeks 3 to 8 a small number of designated residents who were participating in the study. Each staff member was asked to carry out six ten-minute observations per week according to this schedule (a total of 36 observations over the six-week period).

Staff members were instructed to observe residents only in public areas of the home and to ensure they observed them while they were awake. Care staff were advised to position themselves close enough to the residents that they could observe what they were doing but not so close that they were invading their personal space. In addition, staff members were advised to observe residents at different times of the day. As part of their observations, care staff were instructed to interact with residents using a stimulus 'object'. This could be something personal to the resident or an item from the care home. In case such objects were not readily available, care staff were provided with a bag containing examples of stimulus objects: a picture book, a textured cushion and a lavender-filled pillow.

Staff members participated in fortnightly group supervision sessions where they discussed their observations. Individual support was offered weekly between sessions and where staff members were unable to attend scheduled sessions. This gave the staff members an opportunity to discuss any difficulties they were encountering whilst conducting their observations. They were also able to discuss what they had noticed about the residents they were observing. In the final meeting at the end of the intervention period the researchers asked the participating staff about their perceptions of the intervention, and recorded their responses. These responses were later collated and examined to identify common themes. In some cases, responses could be linked to comments made at an earlier stage and recorded in the field notes, demonstrating changes in staff perceptions over the course of the intervention.

As part of their observations the care staff recorded any additional behaviours demonstrated by the residents that were not covered in the AwareCare matrix. This provided an insight into both the care staff members' views on the residents and their increasing recognition of signs of awareness.

Case Study 18.1 – **Sandra**[2]

Sandra was mobile and would often wander around the care home. She could communicate through a few words but was perceived as quiet in comparison to the other residents. She was often found sitting by herself. Through observation it was noted that she was affected by

---

2   All names in case studies in this chapter are pseudonyms.

the high levels of noise and movement in the care home environment and would often go somewhere quiet to get away from it all.

Care worker Cathy noted in one of her observations of Sandra that '[She is] very observant of people around her and who was talking. She was looking at the pictures in the photo album and would point out the pictures she particularly liked.' The observations gave Cathy the opportunity to learn more about Sandra and to notice that Sandra did respond to her surroundings. Using the picture book helped Cathy to interact with Sandra and learn something about her.

Case Study 18.2 – Lois

Lois was immobile and spent much of her day either sitting in a communal room or in her bedroom on bed rest. Through observation it was evident that Lois experienced some discomfort, as she would often move around in her chair in a way that suggested she was in pain. She could say single words but did not tend to interact with the other residents or care staff.

Care worker Kirstin observed Lois and noted that 'Lois held all of the introduced items at the same time but did not want to do much with them. She is very aware of most things going on around her and explores constantly with her eyes when other staff are moving tables/serving drinks/coming into the room/leaving the room. She is a people watcher, very aware of what is going on around her.' By carefully observing Lois it was evident to Kirstin that Lois was acutely aware of what was going on around her, but as this awareness was often only evident in her eye movements it could be easily missed.

Case Study 18.3 – John

John was non-verbal, immobile and unable to sit up independently. John did not appear to interact with the other residents or take an interest in what was going on around him.

Ann noted in one of her observations of John that 'John sat in his chair in the main lounge. John was tired, but when another resident shouted he smiled, looked at him then at me. He smiled and pulled faces.' This again illustrates that through careful observation it was clear that John was making responses to events that were going on around him. As these responses were very subtle they could easily be missed.

Outcomes

Clare *et al.* (2013) found that residents receiving the AwareCare intervention had significantly better quality of life (QUALID: Weiner *et al.* 2000), as rated by family members, than those in the control group, although care staff ratings of quality of life did not change as a result of the intervention. Positive feedback was also provided by the care staff who had taken part in the intervention. First, the training was felt to be informative and educational, and enabled some staff members to feel more effective in their role:

> 'I feel I can do my job better now through learning how to observe individuals.'

> 'I have become more observant towards clients. I have worked in the care sector for 15 years and the training has made me become more aware of things.'

Second, staff found it beneficial to spend one-to-one time with residents in this way as it allowed for greater understanding of their behaviour and responses. Through observation they could learn something 'new' about the residents:

> 'I enjoyed having more one-to-one time with the residents.'

> 'I'm always very busy and so it was nice to have some time with the residents. I have enjoyed having the opportunity to sit and observe residents properly and to be able to pick up on little things about the residents.'

Third, staff who had previously thought that certain residents were non-responsive found that through observation they could detect a range of responses. One staff member, when given her observation schedule during initial training, commented: 'Oh no, I've got to observe [resident] but she doesn't do anything, that's going to be very boring.' At the final meeting at the end of the intervention, the same staff member described how she could now tell that this resident showed awareness:

> 'Well, when I was giving [resident] her breakfast the other morning, she didn't like it…her facial expression, I could tell she wasn't keen.'

Similarly, another staff member who commented initially, 'Oh, I've got a boring one [resident], look', spoke of this resident as follows in the final meeting:

'She does respond… A lot of eye movements and turning her head, and if you suddenly touch her and she hasn't seen you she jumps… She is very aware.'

The 'blinded' researchers also noted positive changes in the intervention homes, whether in the behaviour of participating care staff, the responses of participating residents or in the environment generally. They noted:

'The staff appear to be working more flexibly and trying different techniques.'

'[Member of care staff] appeared to spend more time having conversations with the residents than at baseline. He also appeared to be very sensitive towards the residents' behaviour.'

'[Member of care staff] commented that [resident] is more aware than people think.'

'[Resident] was given a textured cushion and a soft toy to hold… [resident] was given a magazine to hold and look through…when she had the magazine she was more alert.'

Key features needed for implementation

There are challenges in implementing interventions in care home environments. In this study the engagement of care staff and the support from care home managers varied considerably. In order for the intervention to be successful, there needs to be support from the care home manager to ensure that care staff are able take part in the training sessions and have adequate time to conduct their observations. Equally, staff members need to be committed to taking part in the intervention. Some care staff found it difficult to find free time to conduct their observations. Care staff were informed that it was important to let other staff members know that they were conducting their observations so as to prevent them from interrupting them. Observation sessions could be interrupted, for instance by other residents speaking to the care staff or because care staff had to go and help other residents. If this happened, they were advised to record the interruption on their observation form and finish their observation at another time.

The intervention was designed for care staff with a good grasp of the English language, and none of the care staff who took part in the study had any difficulty in completing the form. In addition, in order to take part in the study the staff member needed to be a permanent employee, working 15 hours or more per week, who had been in post for at least two months. This was to try to ensure that participating care staff did not leave their employment at the home during the intervention period. Despite this, five members of care staff were no longer working at the care home by the time of the follow-up assessments. This highlights the frequent transient nature of employment in care settings in the UK and is one of the challenges in providing training to care staff.

It was important that care staff were supported during their initial observations. This could be achieved either by having the researcher sitting in on their first observation or by having the researcher checking their first observation and making sure they had completed the form appropriately. Weekly face-to-face contact with the researcher was also important as it helped motivate the staff to do their observations. Equally, the care staff could speak to the researchers about any difficulties they were having completing the observations, and the researcher would see what they could do to help. Generally care staff needed less support as the weeks went by and they became more experienced in using the measure.

The homes that took part in this study varied in size and resident characteristics. Some were homes specifically for people with dementia, while others also had residents with no cognitive impairment. There were no difficulties in implementing the intervention in the different types of settings. However, residents with no cognitive impairment were a little more inquisitive as to what was going on, so the care staff needed to explain the study to them. In the larger homes, care staff were rotated around the units they worked in, and the researchers needed to work with the care home manager to ensure that the care staff were able to conduct observations with residents in other units.

Conclusion

The AwareCare intervention is an effective way of helping care staff to identify and understand awareness in people with severe dementia. Care staff are able to use the AwareCare measure effectively as a practice tool, and they feel this is useful in enabling them to identify and understand residents' responses. The study has further shown that where this is done, family members perceive an improvement in the quality of life of their relatives. Developing a better understanding of awareness in people with severe dementia has the potential to improve both quality of care and quality of life.

References

Abramowitz, L. (2008) 'Working with advanced dementia patients in a day care setting.' *Journal of Gerontological Social Work 50*, 25–35.

Boller, F., Verny, M., Hugonot-Diener, L. and Saxton, J. (2002) 'Clinical features and assessment of severe dementia: A review.' *European Journal of Neurology 9*, 125–136.

Clare, L. (2010) 'Awareness in people with severe dementia: Review and integration.' *Aging & Mental Health 14*, 20–32.

Clare, L., Woods, R.T., Whitaker, R.,Wilson, B.A. and Downs, M. (2010) 'Development of an awareness-based intervention to enhance quality of life in severe dementia.' *Trials 11*, 73.

Clare, L., Markova, I., Roth, I. and Morris, R. (2011) 'Awareness in Alzheimer's disease and associated dementias: Theoretical framework and clinical implications.' *Aging & Mental Health 15*, 936–944.

Clare, L., Whitaker, R., Quinn, C., Jelley, H. *et al.* (2012) 'AwareCare: Development and validation of an observational measure of awareness in people with severe dementia.' *Neuropsychological Rehabilitation 22*, 113–133.

Clare, L., Whitaker, R., Woods, R.T., Quinn, C. *et al.* (2013) 'AwareCare: A pilot randomized controlled trial of an awareness-based staff training intervention to improve quality of life for residents with severe dementia in long-term care settings.' *International Psychogeriatrics 25*, 1, 128–139.

Ekman, S.L., Norberg, A., Viitanen, M. and Winblad, B. (1991) 'Care of demented patients with severe communication problems.' *Scandinavian Journal of Caring Sciences 5*, 163–170.

Hansebo, G. and Kihlgren, M. (2002) 'Carers' interactions with patients suffering from severe dementia: A difficult balance to facilitate mutual togetherness.' *Journal of Clinical Nursing 11*, 225–236.

Lawton, M.P., Van Haitsma, K. and Klapper, J. (1996) 'Observed affect in nursing home residents with Alzheimer's disease.' *Journals of Gerontology B 51*, 3–14.

Magai, C., Cohen, C., Gomberg, D., Malatesta, C. and Culver, C. (1996) 'Emotional expression during mid- to late-stage dementia.' *International Psychogeriatrics 8*, 383–395.

Quinn, C., Clare, L., Jelley, H., Bruce, E. and Woods, B. (2013) '"It's in the eyes": How family members and care staff understand awareness in people with severe dementia.' *Aging & Mental Health 18*, 2, 260–268.

Reisberg, B. (1988) 'Functional Assessment Staging (FAST).' *Psychopharmacology Bulletin 24*, 653–659.

Shiel, A., Horn, S.A., Wilson, B.A., McLellan, D.L., Watson, M.J. and Campbell, M. (2000) 'The Wessex Head Injury Matrix (WHIM) main scale: A preliminary report on a scale to assess and monitor patient recovery after severe head injury.' *Clinical Rehabilitation 14*, 408–416.

Weiner, M.F., Martin-Cook, K., Svetlik, D.A., Saine, K., Foster, B. and Fontaine, C.S. (2000) 'The Quality of Life in Late-Stage Dementia (QUALID) Scale.' *Journal of the American Medical Directors' Association 1*, 114–116.

Wilson, B.A., Shiel, A., McLellan, L., Horn, S. and Watson, M.A. (2001) 'Monitoring recovery of cognitive function following severe brain injury.' *Brain Impairment 2*, 22–28.

About the Contributors

Elisa Aguirre is a researcher at the Division of Psychology and Language Sciences, University College London, UK.

Stefanie Auer is Professor at the Faculty of Health and Medicine, Department for Clinical Neurosciences and Preventive Medicine, Danube-University, Krems, Austria.

Kevin Charras is Head of the Training Center and the Living lab at the Fondation Médéric Alzheime, Paris, France.

Linda Clare is Professor of Clinical Psychology of Ageing and Dementia and Director of the Centre for Research in Ageing and Cognitive Health (REACH), a joint venture between the School of Psychology and the Medical School at the University of Exeter, UK.

Rabih Chattat is Associate Professor of Clinical Psychology at the University of Bologna, Italy.

Irena Draskovic worked as a senior researcher at Radboud University Nijmegen Medical Center, Nijmegen, the Netherlands.

Rose Marie Drőes is Professor of Psychosocial Care for People with Dementia at the Department of Psychiatry, VU University Medical Centre, Amsterdam, the Netherlands.

Ane Eckermann is a nurse who worked at the Danish Dementia Research Centre, Copenhagen University Hospital in Denmark and is now Head of Projects and Development Management at the Danish Alzheimer's Association.

Suzannah Evans was a Research Occupational Therapist (OT) who delivered the Cognitive Rehabilitation Intervention for both the pilot and definitive GREAT Trial, whist employed by Health and Care Research Wales. She now works as a specialist OT for the Betsi Cadwaladr University Health Board, North Wales, UK.

Debby Gerritsen is Professor of Well-being in Long-term Care at the Radboud University Medical Center in Radboud University in Nijmegen, the Netherlands.

Marie Gianelli (now retired) was Associate Professor (Psychology) at the Faculty of Medicine and Surgery, University of Genova, Italy.

Dana Hradcová is an ethicist and care consultant at the Centre of Expertise in Longevity and Long Term Care (CELLO), Charles University, Prague, Czech Republic.

Iva Holmerová is a consultant geriatrician, Associate Professor, and Head of the Centre of Expertise in Longevity and Long Term Care (CELLO), Faculty of Humanities at Charles University, Prague, Czech Republic. She is also chairperson of the Alzheimer's Europe Board.

Hein van Hout is a psychologist and Associate Professor at the Department of General Practice and Elderly Care Medicine at Vrije University in Amsterdam, the Netherlands.

Karlijn Joling is a senior researcher at the Department of General Practice and Elderly Care Medicine, VU University Medical Centre, EMGO, Amsterdam, the Netherlands.

Aleksandra (Ola) Kudlicka is a senior research fellow at the Centre for Research in Ageing and Cognitive Health (REACH), University of Exeter, UK.

Alexander Kurz is Professor and Head of the Centre for Cognitive Disorders at the Department of Psychiatry and Psychotherapy, at the Technische Universität München, Munich, Germany.

Ruslan Leontjevas is Assistant Professor in Psychodiagnostics at the Open University in Eindhoven, the Netherlands.

Jill Manthorpe is Professor of Social Work and Director of the NIHR Policy Research Unit on Health and Social Care Workforce at King's College London, UK. She has longstanding interests in policy and practice in dementia care and is a member of INTERDEM.

Franka Meiland is a health psychologist and senior researcher at the Department of Elderly Care Medicine, and lecturer at Gerion of Amsterdam University Medical Centers, location VUmc, Amsterdam, the Netherlands.

Esme Moniz-Cook is Professor of Clinical Psychology, Ageing and Dementia Care at the Faculty of Health Sciences, University of Hull, UK. She has worked for over 30 years in dementia care research and clinical practice with longstanding interest in developing and translating dementia care research into practice. In 1999 she founded INTERDEM, a multidisciplinary network of psychosocial intervention applied dementia care research (www.interdem.org).

Gail Mountain is an occupational therapist and is Professor of Applied Dementia Research and Director of the Centre for Applied Dementia Studies at the University of Bradford, UK.

Martin Orrell is Professor and Director of the Institute of Mental Health and Head of the Division of Psychiatry and Applied Psychology in the Faculty of Medicine and Health Sciences at the University of Nottingham, UK.

Catherine Quinn is a lecturer in dementia studies at the Centre for Applied Dementia Studies, University of Bradford, UK.

Alfredo Raglio coordinates the Master's in Music Therapy at the Department of Public Health, University of Pavia, Italy and works at the Istituti Clinici Scientifici Maugeri IRCCS Pavia, Italy and at the Fondazione Istituto Ospedaliero di Sospiro, Cremona, Italy.

Chris Rewston is a clinical psychologist at the Hull Memory Clinic, Humber NHS Teaching Foundation Trust, Hull, UK.

Henriëtte van der Roest is Head of the Program on Aging at the Trimbos Institute, Utrecht, the Netherlands. She previously worked as researcher in dementia at the Department of General Practice and Elderly Care Medicine, Amsterdam UMC, Vrije Universiteit Amsterdam, the Netherlands, and in dementia research in the UK.

Sarah Kate Smith is a researcher at the Institute for Dementia in the University of Salford, UK, and has previously worked at the Universities of Sheffield and Bradford.

Aimee Spector is Professor of Old Age Clinical Psychology, Division of Psychology and Language Sciences at University College London, UK.

Michal Šteffl is Head of the Department of Physiology and Biochemistry at Charles University in Prague, Czech Republic.

Amy Streater is a senior researcher at North East London NHS Foundation Trust and the Division of Psychology and Language Sciences, University College London, UK.

Michal Synek is a sociology graduate and works at the Center of Expertise in Longevity and Long Term Care (CELLO), Charles University, Prague, Czech Republic.

Angelika Thöne-Otto is a senior clinical neuropsychologist and group leader at the Clinic for Cognitive Neurology, University of Leipzig, Germany.

Johanne Tonga is a psychologist at the Frambu Resource Centre for Rare Disorders in Siggerud, Norway. Her dementia research was at the memory clinic, Oslo University Hospital (Ullevål) and the Department of Old Age Psychiatry, Oslo University Hospital (Gaustad), Norway.

Ingun Ulstein is an old age psychiatrist at the Memory Clinic, Department of Geriatric Medicine, Ullevål, Oslo University Hospital, Norway.

Hana Vaňková is a geriatrician at the Centre of Gerontology, researcher at CELLO Faculty of Humanities and Assistant Professor (Geriatrics) of the Third Faculty of Medicine, Charles University, Prague, Czech Republic.

Petr Veleta is a kinanthropologist working at the Opera, National Theatre, Prague, Czech Republic.

Gunhild Waldemar is a neurologist, Professor and Director of the Danish Dementia Research Centre at the University of Copenhagen, Denmark.

Katja Werheid is a clinical psychologist/neuropsychologist, Associate Professor at the Department of Psychology at Humboldt University of Berlin, Germany, and Head of the Neuropsychology Unit at Klinikum Ernst von Bergmann (Potsdam), Germany.

Jitka Zgola is a retired occupational therapist. She now contributes to the field through consultancy and as an author, educator and advisor to those who care for people living with Alzheimer's disease and related disorders.

Sytse Zuidema is an elderly care physician and Professor of Elderly Care Medicine and Dementia at the University Medical Center, Department of General Practice and Elderly Care Medicine, University of Groningen, the Netherlands.

Subject Index

Author Index

Pearce, W. 30
Peavy, V.R. 49, 50
Pei, J-J. 100
Peisah, C. 43
Penna, A. 73
Pepin, R. 31
Peterson, C.B. 146
Philpin, S. 244
Phinney, A. 100, 101, 103, 104
Phung, K.T.T. 49, 62
Pierzchala, A. 155
Pini, S. 31
Pinquart, M. 151, 160
Pols, J. 249
Potter, R. 107
Poulos, C.J. 13
Pozzi, C. 31
Price, K. 19
Projekt GOS 199
Purandare, N. 224

Quin, R. 105
Quinn, C. 261

Raglio, A. 179, 180, 181, 186
Rahman, S. 24
Raia, P. 220
Raman, S. 30
Ranganath, C. 227
Rapoport, A. 225
Ravelin, T. 193
Reddecliff, L. 106
Reese, M. 168
Reid, D. 105
Reisberg, B. 75, 262
Ridder, H.M. 182, 187
Rio, R. 187
Robert, P. 209
Roberts, E. 244
Robinson, L. 107
Rockwood, K. 115
Rodin, J. 222
Rogers, A. 33
Röhricht, F. 191
Rollnick, S. 123
Rosler, A. 191, 193
Rösner, M. 235
Rowlands, J.M. 105

Royal College of Psychiatrists 31
Ryan, N.P. 31, 43
Rylatt, P. 197

Sabat, S.R. 101, 102
Sachs, O. 25
Sader, A. 244
Sæteren, B. 167
Samsi, K. 24
Sandman, P.O. 235
Santos, R. 180
Särkämö, T. 187, 188
Schell, E. 246
Schultz, H. 76
Schultz, R. 222
Schwarzer, R. 134
SCIE 21, 24
Scottish Government 166
Selbaek, G. 204
Sellick, J. 79
Sharma, S. 13
Shiel, A. 262
Sipos, I. 73, 74
Smalbrugge, M. 204
Smith, L. 191
Smith, S.K. 108
Smits, C.H.M. 66, 101
Søgaard. R. 53
Sommerlad, A. 168
Song, J.A. 166
Sørensen, L.V. 59, 101, 104
Sorensen, S. 151, 160
Sousa, L. 43
Span, E. 75
Span, M. 145
Spector, A. 85, 86, 87, 90, 91, 93, 95, 96
Starkstein, S.E. 126
Stephan, I. 195
Stewart, R. 234
Stollmeijer, A. 244
Streater, A. 94
Streiner, D.L. 31
Stuss, D.T. 204
Suchá, J. 193
Surr, C.A. 9
Sutin, A.R. 13
Swaffer, K. 9, 10, 21, 24
Synek, M. 256
Szczesniak, D. 69, 81